C000231906

VASCULAR COMPLICA~~~~~~~~~~~
CURRENT ISSUES IN PATHOGENESIS AND TREATMENT

Editor **Richard Donnelly** MD, PhD, FRCP, FRACP
Division of Vascular Medicine
University of Nottingham
Derbyshire Royal Infirmary
UK

Associate Editor **Jost Jonas** MD
Faculty for Clinical Medicine
University Eye Clinic
Mannheim
Germany

Blackwell
Science

© 2002 by Blackwell Science Ltd
a Blackwell Publishing Company

EDITORIAL OFFICES:
Osney Mead, Oxford OX2 0EL, UK
   Tel: +44 (0)1865 206206
108 Cowley Road, Oxford OX4 1JF, UK
   Tel: +44 (0)1865 791100
Blackwell Publishing USA, 350 Main Street, Malden, MA 02148-5018, USA
   Tel: +1 781 388 8250
Iowa State Press, a Blackwell Publishing Company, 2121 State Avenue, Ames, Iowa 50014-8300, USA
   Tel: +1 515 292 0140
Blackwell Munksgaard, Nørre Søgade 35, PO Box 2148, Copenhagen, DK-1016, Denmark
   Tel: +45 77 33 33 33
Blackwell Publishing Asia, 54 University Street, Carlton, Victoria 3053, Australia
   Tel: +61 (0)3 9347 0300
Blackwell Verlag, Kurfürstendamm 57, 10707 Berlin, Germany
   Tel: +49 (0)30 32 79 060
Blackwell Publishing, 10 rue Casimir Delavigne, 75006 Paris, France
   Tel: +33 1 53 10 33 10

The right of the Author to be identified as the Author of this Work has been asserted in accordance with the Copyright, Designs and Patents Act 1988.

All rights reserved. No part of this publication may be reproduced, stored in a retrieval system, or transmitted, in any form or by any means, electronic, mechanical, photocopying, recording or otherwise, except as permitted by the UK Copyright, Designs and Patents Act 1988, without the prior permission of the publisher.

The Blackwell Publishing logo is a trade mark of Blackwell Publishing Ltd

First published 2002

Catalogue records for this title are available from the British Library and Library of Congress

ISBN 0-632-06513-3

Set in 9.5/12pt Branding Serif
Text layout and design by Designers Collective Limited
Printed and bound in Great Britain by Ashford Colour Press Ltd, Gosport, Hants

For further information on Blackwell Publishing, visit our website:
www.blackwell-science.com

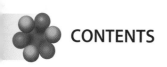

CONTENTS

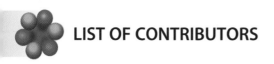 **LIST OF CONTRIBUTORS**

Hean-Choon Chen FRCS, FRCOpath
Consultant Ophthalmologist
Derbyshire Royal Infirmary
Derby, UK

Richard Donnelly MD, PhD, FRCP, FRACP
Professor of Vascular Medicine
University of Nottingham
and Honorary Consultant Physician
J. O'Neil Diabetic Centre
Derbyshire Royal Infirmary
Derby, UK

Adrian R. Scott MD, FRCP
Consultant Physician
J. O'Neil Diabetic Centre
Derbyshire Royal Infirmary
Derby, UK

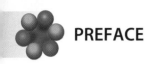

PREFACE

Diabetes affects over 100 million people worldwide, and the relentless progression of diabetic vascular complications results in disabling, multisystem morbidities, e.g. blindness, dialysis and amputation; the associated healthcare expenditure is enormous and patients with diabetes have a reduced life expectancy. Diabetic retinopathy is the leading cause of blindness in people of working age, but there is heightened clinical anticipation that blocking protein kinase C (PKC) activation–a major pathway in glycaemic vascular injury–may ameliorate diabetic eye disease as an adjunct to existing glucose- and blood pressure-lowering strategies.

This book is aimed at healthcare professionals involved in the clinical management of diabetic complications, especially retinopathy, and is divided into three major sections: (I) an overview of the clinical features and evidence-based therapies for microvascular and macrovascular disease; (II) a detailed review of diabetic retinopathy with an emphasis on diagnosis and treatment of maculopathy, the principal cause of blindness in patients with type 2 diabetes; and (III) a simplified description of the biochemical pathways involved in hyperglycaemia-induced structural and functional vascular abnormalities, in particular the emergence of PKC as a new therapeutic target for delaying and reversing important pathological changes in retinal, renal and endothelial tissues.

Richard Donnelly

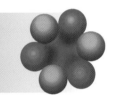

SECTION I

MICRO- AND MACROVASCULAR COMPLICATIONS OF DIABETES

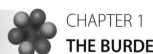

INTRODUCTION

The 21st century will see diabetes emerge as the world's commonest chronic disease. Whilst the bulk of this will be type 2 diabetes (90%) the incidence has been rising in both types.

The direct and indirect costs of diabetes and its complications, plus the associated reduction in quality and quantity of life, will have considerable economic consequences. These effects will be most noticeable in developing countries which are going to see a disproportionate increase in the prevalence of diabetes over the next few decades. It has been estimated that the world-wide prevalence of diabetes will double between 1990 and 2010. Epidemiological studies in the USA have shown that the number of people with known diabetes has increased from around 1.5 million in 1958 to 10.5 million in 1998. Most states in the USA report a prevalence of over 8% and this fails to take into account those people with undiagnosed diabetes. Most screening studies indicate that at least 50% of people found to have diabetes were silently undiagnosed for sometime.

THE NATURAL HISTORY OF TYPE 1 DIABETES

Although onset is predominantly in childhood or young adulthood, a significant proportion will be diagnosed over the age of 30 years. The peak ages for onset, however, are around puberty and between 4 and 6 years old. Life expectancy is reduced, though there is some evidence that this is improving.

The British Diabetic Association Cohort study (1972–93), a prospective follow-up of insulin-treated patients with diabetes diagnosed under the age of 30 years, showed increased mortality at all ages. Avoidable metabolic complications such as hypoglycaemia and diabetic ketoacidosis accounted for most of the excess mortality among those under 30 years but after 20 years of diabetes the impact of atherosclerotic macrovascular complications steadily increases. The prognosis is particularly disturbing for children diagnosed with type 1 diabetes under the age of 10 years; previous reports have indicated that 60% were dead within 40 years of diagnosis. With increasing duration of diabetes, the prevalence of retinopathy, nephropathy and neuropathy is highest in those with poor glycaemic control and lowest in those with good control. The Diabetes Control and Complications Trial (DCCT 1995) established quite clearly that good glycaemic control in type 1 diabetes can reduce the incidence and progression of microvascular complications but the risk of a vascular event increases with duration of diabetes and the presence of nephropathy. DCCT was under-powered, and the patients too young, to be sure if improved glycaemia reduced the risk of macrovascular complications but the trend was for good control to be associated with a reduction in vascular events.

EPIDEMIOLOGY OF TYPE 1 DIABETES

The worldwide variation in incidence of type 1 diabetes is considerable though the pattern of presentation is similar. The incidence is showing signs of increasing at all ages but most noticeably in the under 5's. In under 16's, northern Europe (Finland, Scotland and Sweden) has the highest rates with up to 30–35 cases per 100 000 of the population aged <16 years per year. Japan, China and Korea have rates that are as low as 0.5–2 cases per 100 000 per year. It is tempting to think that this is due mainly to genetic differences but there are different incidences in genetically similar countries such as Norway and Iceland, suggesting that environmental factors have a very significant influence. Whilst the pathophysiology of islet cell destruction has been well defined, the trigger for this process remains uncertain. Despite the relatively sudden onset of symptoms, family studies have shown there is a long pro-dromal period of immune activation. Viruses and cows milk protein are currently the main contenders that may initiate this process in the genetically susceptible.

THE NATURAL HISTORY OF TYPE 2 DIABETES

It is well recognized that patients with type 2 diabetes often have established complications at the time of diagnosis. In the UK Prospective Diabetes Study (UKPDS), for example, 36% of newly diagnosed patients had retinopathy, 12% neuropathy and 2% proteinuria at recruitment. This may well be an underestimate, because in UKPDS patients with established vascular disease or retinopathy requiring laser therapy were excluded. Using prospective studies which have studied the rate of progression of retinopathy, it is estimated that at diagnosis of type 2 diabetes, patients are likely to have had their diabetes for between 8 and 12 years and, prior to diabetes, impaired glucose tolerance for very much longer. Death from ischaemic heart disease, stroke or lower extremity ischaemia occurs in over 60% of patients.

EPIDEMIOLOGY OF TYPE 2 DIABETES

Although there is good evidence that type 2 diabetes is a heterogeneous condition with a number of genetic subgroups, the current view supports the idea that for the majority of people this is a metabolic disorder in the genetically susceptible, precipitated by lifestyle changes which have led to a sedentary lifestyle and obesity. Essentially it is a failure of adaptation to a new environment which has changed in the course of a few generations. Elliot Joslin went to study the Pima Indians at the start of the 20th century because of their low prevalence of diabetes. By the end of the century they ranked alongside the Pacific Micronesians from Nauru for having the highest prevalence of type 2 diabetes in the world.

The 'thrifty gene' hypothesis postulates that humans evolving in a harsh environment, where famine and high physical activity was the norm, may have developed fuel efficient systems, which, when faced with limitless supplies of food and a sedentary lifestyle, leads to the metabolic disturbances now characterized as the metabolic syndrome (central obesity, hypertension, hyperlipidaemia and glucose intolerance). Underlying this is insulin resistance, which partly relates to fat distribution—the greater the proportion of intra-abdominal fat compared to the total, the greater the degree of insulin resistance. The distribution of fat deposition is genetically determined and there is evidence that there are ethnic differences in body composition. Insulin sensitivity studies suggest that despite matching for age and body mass index (BMI), significant differences persist between ethnic groups which may explain the wide variations in prevalence of type 2 diabetes across the world. Nauruans and Pimas have already been mentioned, but other high-risk groups include South Indians, native American Indians, Mexican Americans and African Americans, all of whom have a higher prevalence of diabetes than Whites. This is despite the epidemic of obesity which effects all ethnic groups in the developed world. There is also an inverse relationship with poverty, but this is insufficient to explain all the population differences in prevalence.

The prevalence of type 2 diabetes is similar in men and women but increases with age. The best studied populations are in the USA (**Fig. 1.1**) and recent data suggests that diagnosed diabetes is most prevalent in the middle-aged and elderly (**Table 1.1**). The incidence is increasing in childhood and is related to obesity.

THE COST OF DIABETES

There is considerable morbidity associated with diabetes and calculating the cost can at best be an imprecise estimate. Diabetes is the leading cause of blindness, end-stage renal failure (ESRF) and lower-extremity amputation (LEA) in the developed world. People with diabetes experience high rates of macrovascular complications at least twice that of non-diabetics.

In the UK, estimates of the cost of diabetes were first attempted in 1989 using 1984 data and this suggested that 4–5% of all UK healthcare expenditure went on people with diabetes. More recent data suggest the figure is closer to

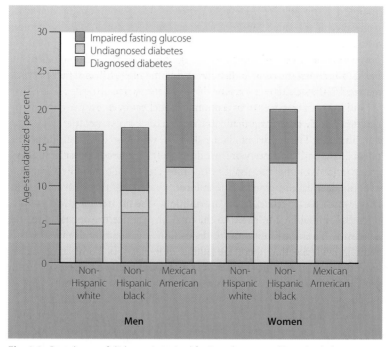

Fig. 1.1 Prevalence of diabetes, impaired fasting glucose, and impaired glucose tolerance in US adults.From the Third National Health and Nutrition Examination Survey 1988–94, *Diabetes Care* 1998; **21**: 518–524.

Prevalence of diabetes by age in USA	
Age (years)	Prevalence of known diabetes (%)
18–44	1.5
45–64	6
Over 65	11

Table 1.1 Prevalence of diabetes by age in USA.

8%, and that one-third of total expenditure on diabetes is spent on those aged zero to 24 years. The difficulties, however, are that it is difficult to cost episodes in patients with multiple pathologies and coding has been shown to under-record secondary diagnoses such as diabetes. Most economic assessments concentrate on direct costs, although clearly indirect costs, such as time off work, and intangible costs, such as lost productivity, will inflate the figures considerably.

Surveys from the USA suggest that healthcare expenditure was over $11,000 per year per person with diabetes compared to $2,600 for people without diabetes. Over 60% was due to inpatient hospitalization.

Nevertheless, there are effective strategies for the prevention or delay of complications associated with diabetes and both the DCCT in type 1 diabetes and the UKPDS in type 2 diabetes have demonstrated the effectiveness of intensification of treatment. An economic model has been used to analyse the costs of DCCT, enabling calculation of the costs of preventing end-stage complications. The model predicted that intensive therapy would result in approximately 15 years free from the first major complications of type 1 diabetes and additional years of life free from blindness, ESRF and LEA (**Fig. 1.2**). It was projected that intensive therapy would prolong life by about 5 years and the cost was approximately $29,000 per year of life gained.

Similar economic modelling has looked at the cost-effectiveness of 'comprehensive' or intensive care of type 2 diabetes (**Table 1.2**). Such models are predicting the likelihood of complications developing in a diabetic population. One such model suggests that with standard care (non-intensive) over a life time, 19% of subjects would become blind, 17% would develop ESRF and 16% would require LEA . With intensification of glucose control these figures could be reduced by up to 75% (but with no effect on cardiovascular outcome) with increased survival of 1.3 years. The average life-time cost was

Predicted reduction in life time costs of end-stage complications through comprehensive care for type 2 diabetes			
Cost elements	Standard care	Comprehensive care	Difference
Present value costs (3% discount rate)			
General and diabetes-related medical care ($)	32,365	58,312	25,947
Eye disease ($)	3,128	1,536	(1,592)
Renal disease ($)	9,437	960	(8,477)
Neuropathy/lower-extremity amputations ($)	4,381	1,469	(2,912)
New coronary heart disease ($)	13,458	14,414	956
Total costs ($)	62,769	76,922	13,922
QALY (undiscounted)	16.04	18.03	1.9
QALY (discounted 3%)	11.43	12.30	0.87
Life-years (undiscounted)	17.05	18.37	1.32
Incremental cost/QALY gained	—	—	16,002

Table 1.2 Predicted reduction in life time costs of end-stage complications through comprehensive care for type 2 diabetes. Data are averages per person per life time. Cost savings are indicated in parentheses.

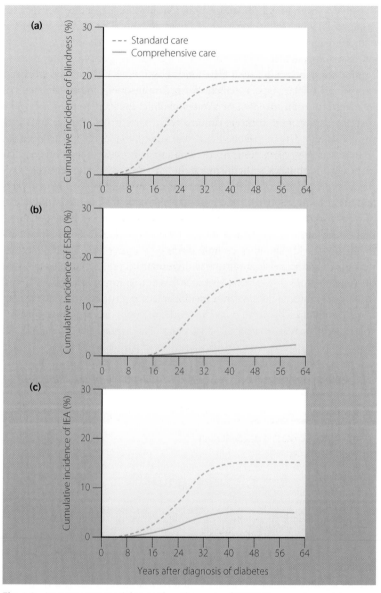

Fig. 1.2 An economic model to analyse the costs of DCCT. For people receiving standard care, the model predicts sharply increasing cumulative incidence of complications, including: (a) blindness, (b) ESRD, and (c) lower-extremity amputation (LEA) with increasing duration of type 2 diabetes. The model predicted a substantially lower incidence of these long-term complications with a program of comprehensive care. *Diabetes Care* 1998; **21** (Suppl 3): C19–C24.

$40,000 more than with standard care. Of course, these models are limited because they have only looked at the cost and benefits of intensification of glycaemic control and clearly there are many other interventions available to reduce macrovascular risk.

These somewhat daunting economic assessments of diabetes care can be viewed from different perspectives. For politicians and public health specialists, it provides an incentive to invest now in primary prevention of type 2 diabetes, as treatment costs are unsustainable, given the epidemic of diabetes that is sweeping the developed and developing worlds. For clinicians, the challenge is to develop cost-effective strategies and deliver high-quality diabetes services that reach the many rather than the few. Comprehensive eye-screening, ensuring everyone at high vascular risk receives low-dose aspirin and annual foot assessments are examples of affordable interventions with proven benefits, but which are not made available to all people with diabetes even in the more affluent societies. For people working in the pharmaceutical industry, they must not forget that they remain part of the society in which they operate and have a social responsibility. Their challenge is to develop and market safe therapies which generate enough profit to encourage future shareholders to invest, but are not so expensive that only the wealthy can afford them.

CURRENT ISSUES

· Population screening for type 2 diabetes is not widespread and may not be cost-effective but targeted opportunistic screening of high-risk individuals (such as women with prior gestational diabetes, first degree relatives, high-risk ethnic groups, the obese) will identify 70% of those with undiagnosed diabetes.

· A recent randomized controlled study from Finland demonstrates that interventions such as weight loss and exercise programs in patients with impaired glucose tolerance have a role in delaying or preventing the progression to frank diabetes. Studies of the early use of insulin sensitizers in impaired glucose tolerance (IGT) are ongoing.

· The epidemic of obesity affects all ages and consequently the emergence of type 2 diabetes in childhood is increasingly apparent. The prognosis is likely to be particularly bad in this age group and a high incidence of nephropathy and early onset cardiovascular disease is to be expected in South Indians and indigenous Indian populations.

FURTHER READING

DCCT Research Group. Resource utilization and costs of care in the DCCT. *Diabetes Care* 1995; **18**: 1468–1478.

Haffner SM, Stern MP, Hazuda HP, Pugh JA, Patterson JK. Hyperinsulinaemia in a population at high risk for non-insulin dependent diabetes mellitus. *N Engl J Med* 1986; **315**: 220–224.

Rubin RJ, Altman WM, Mendelson DN. Health care expenditures for people with diabetes mellitus, 1992. *J Clin Endocrinol Metab* 1994; **78**: 809A–809F.

The Worldwide Burden of Diabetes. Proceedings of a Workshop. Phoenix, Arizona, USA. *Diabetes Care* 1998; **21**: Suppl 3.

Tuomilehto J, Linström J, Eriksson JG *et al.* Prevention of type 2 diabetes mellitus by changes in lifestyle among subjects with impaired glucose tolerance. *N Engl J Med* 2001; **344**: 1343–50.

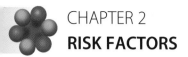
INTRODUCTION

Prior to the use of glycosylation products such as glycosylated haemoglobin and fructosamine in the late 1970s, estimates of glucose control relied on self-reported urine tests, random blood sugars measured in the outpatient setting and other surrogate measures such as frequency of hypoglycaemia, or measurement of 24-hour urinary glucose excretion. Despite these difficulties, the association between duration of diabetes, the degree of hyperglycaemia and the severity of microvascular and neuropathic complications had long been observed in both type 1 and type 2 diabetes. It was also clear that the relationship between glycaemic control and macrovascular disease was not straight forward since people with mild degrees of hyperglycaemia such as those with impaired glucose tolerance had twice the risk of developing coronary heart disease compared to those with normal glucose tolerance. In addition, the association of diabetes (particularly type 2) with multiple vascular risk factors such as hypertension and dyslipidaemia was apparent but it has taken until this last decade or so to realize that it is the interaction of these factors that so alters risk and that each must be viewed in this context, not in isolation. This chapter looks at the influence of hyperglycaemia and other factors on the development of microvascular and macrovascular complications.

HYPERGLYCAEMIA

In a prospective personal series of 4400 patients with diabetes, observed between 1947 and 1973, Pirart showed that poor glycaemic control was clearly related to a higher prevalence of retinopathy, nephropathy and neuropathy compared with patients with better control. With the discovery of glycosylated haemoglobin, the association between long-term hyperglycaemia and complications was confirmed. Retinopathy and microalbuminuria are good markers of microvascular disease and indicative of a generalized vasculopathy. The numerous studies that have looked at the relationship between glycaemic control and both the onset and progression of microvascular complications have produced remarkably consistent results. For example, The Berlin Retinopathy Study was an observational report on children and adolescents with type 1 diabetes who were followed between 1977 and 1993. During that period most young people with type 1 diabetes were followed up by a single centre. Glycosylated haemoglobin (HbA1$_C$) was available from 1980 onwards and urine was tested for microalbumin from 1987 onwards. Data has been published on 346 patients (190 males) who were followed up to the age of 18–22 years. The rate of onset of background retinopathy rose with increasing

HbA1$_C$ from 0.7 events per 100 patient years in the group with a long-term HbA1$_C$ of <7% to 7.3 events per 100 patient years when the long-term HbA1$_C$ was >11%. The incidence of retinopathy increased steeply when the HbA1$_C$ was above 9% (**Fig. 2.1**) and was similar to the results seen in the Diabetes Control and Complications Trial (DCCT).

Surprisingly, glycaemic control did not appear to influence the time to development of retinopathy, except in those with very poor control (HbA1$_C$ > 13%). In all other groups the median time to onset of background diabetic retinopathy was approximately 12 years. Patients with microalbuminuria, however, developed retinopathy after a mean of 11.5 years compared to 14.7 years in those with normoalbuminuria. The chance of remaining free from background retinopathy after 12 years was <25% in patients with microalbuminuria compared to 81% in patients without microalbuminuria.

In the DCCT study, 1441 highly selected patients aged 13–39 years were randomly assigned to intensive or conventional treatment. Approximately half of those randomized had been selected as free of retinopathy and with normal urinary albumin excretion. The other half had mild to moderate retinopathy and urine albumin excretion <200 mg per 24 hours; this group

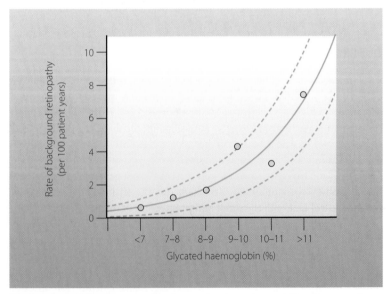

Fig. 2.1   Rate of development of background retinopathy per 100 patient years in different classes of HbA1$_c$. Berlin Retinopathy Study. *Diabetes Care* 1994; **17**(12): 1390–6.

was similarly randomized into a secondary intervention arm. The intensively treated group sustained a 2% drop in HbA1$_C$ to 7%, but glycaemic control remained virtually unchanged in the conventional group (approximately 9% at baseline). There was a 76% adjusted mean risk reduction in the primary prevention arm for the development of retinopathy. In the secondary prevention arm the estimated risk reduction was 54% by intensive treatment.

The Wisconsin Epidemiological Study of Diabetic Retinopathy (WESDR) followed a large population of people with diabetes who were living in southern Wisconsin in the USA from 1979 to 1980. There were around 1200 type 1 diabetics originally diagnosed under the age of 30 and nearly 1800 older onset patients who were predominately type 2 but around of 800 of whom were treated with insulin. Approximately 1300 of this study population were followed up at 10 years—the main reason for the dropout was death before 10 years.

The incidence of retinopathy progression, progression to proliferative retinopathy and incidence of macula oedema increased from the lowest to the higher quartile of HbA1$_C$. For a given level of HbA1$_C$ there were few differences in incidence or progression of retinopathy among the three groups (young type 1, older-onset patients on insulin, older-onset patients on tablets); in addition, there was no evidence of a threshold effect (**Figs 2.2 and 2.3**). The study group examined whether a change in glycaemic control was associated with a change in the risk of progression of retinopathy at 10 years and using mathematical modelling estimated that a 1.5% decrease in HbA1$_C$

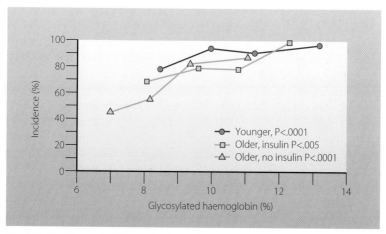

Fig. 2.2 The 10-year incidence of retinopathy by quartile of HbA1$_C$ at baseline in younger-onset group taking insulin, the older group taking insulin, and the older-onset group not taking insulin in WESDR. *Diabetes Care* 1995; **18**: 258–68.

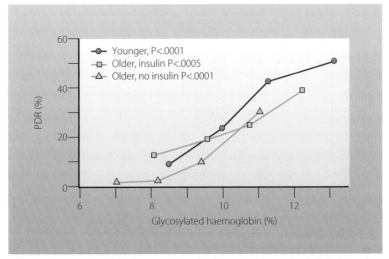

Fig. 2.3 The 10-year progression to proliferative diabetic retinopathy (PDR) by quartile of HbA1$_C$ at baseline in the younger-onset group taking insulin, and the older-onset group taking insulin, and the older-onset group not taking insulin in the WESDR. *Diabetes Care* 1995; **18**: 258–68.

from baseline to 4-year follow-up would be expected to lead to a 33% decease in the 10-year incidence of proliferative retinopathy in the younger age group. A similar fall in HbA1$_C$ produced a 24–40% decrease in incidence in the older age group. The 10-year incidence of proteinuria and renal failure was 28.3 and 7.1% in the younger group and 36.5 and 1.8% in the older onset group. Once again there was a relationship between HbA1$_C$ and the incidence of nephropathy (**Fig. 2.4**).

The WESDR also indicated a relationship between hyperglycaemia and macrovascular disease. There was an increased risk of amputation in both younger and older groups and HbA1$_C$ was associated with increased risk of death. After correction for age and sex the hazard ratio of dying for the fourth quartile of HbA1$_C$ compared to the first quartile of HbA1$_C$ was 1.9%. In the older group, for example, the 10-year survival in the lowest quartile of HbA1$_C$ was 62.8% compared with 41.7% of those in the highest quartile (**Fig. 2.5**).

Interestingly, in WESDR 29% of younger onset patients and 43% of older onset patients did not manifest proliferative diabetic retinopathy (PDR) or proteinuria despite being in the third or fourth quartile of hyperglycaemia. This raises the possibility that some patients are 'protected' from complications or that others are more susceptible. A number of studies of patients

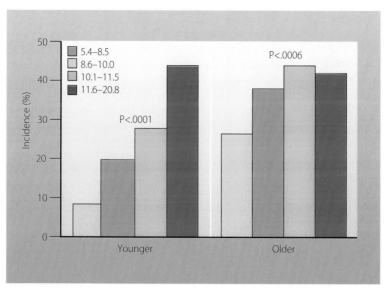

Fig. 2.4   The incidence of gross proteinuria in people with insulin-dependent diabetes mellitus by quartile of HbA1$_c$. *Diabetes Care* 1995; **18**: 258–68.

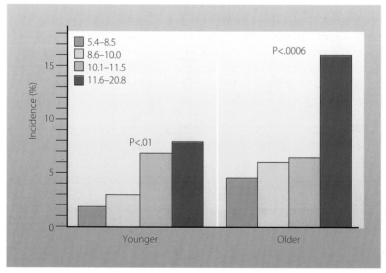

Fig. 2.5   The 10-year incidence of lower extremity amputation by quartile of HbA1$_c$ at baseline, in the younger and older onset groups participating in the WESDR. *Diabetes Care* 1995; **18**: 258–68.

with type 1 diabetes have suggested that as many as 20% of patients do not develop microvascular complications even as late as 30–40 years after the onset of the disease. On the other hand, a small minority may have severe retinopathy after only 5–7 years. Clustering of nephropathy, for example, has been observed in some families and the history of essential hypertension in a first-degree relative is associated with an increased risk of nephropathy in the family member with type 1 diabetes. In WESDR there were no obvious differences between people with type 1 and type 2 diabetes in the incidence of microvascular complications in relation to rising HbA1$_C$.

In the UK Prospective Diabetes Study (UKPDS) the risk of each of the microvascular and macrovascular complications of type 2 diabetes was strongly associated with hyperglycaemia, as measured by HbA1$_C$. There was no evidence of a threshold and there was a threefold increase over the range of <6% to ≥10% (**Fig. 2.6**).

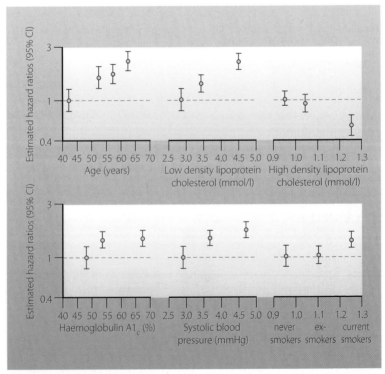

Fig. 2.6 Estimated hazard ratios for significant risk factors for coronary artery disease occurring in 335 out of 3055 diabetic patients. *BMJ* 1998; **316**: 823–8, with permission.

HYPERTENSION, HYPERLIPIDAEMIA AND SMOKING

Hypertension exacerbates the micro- and macrovascular complications of diabetes (**Fig. 2.7**) but it is important to differentiate between the hypertension associated with the two main types of diabetes. People with type 1 diabetes at diagnosis have similar blood pressures to non-diabetics and the development of hypertension increases with diabetes duration and is associated with the development of nephropathy. Microalbuminuria and proteinuria are manifestations of renal involvement. Untreated, the hypertension worsens, protein excretion rates increase and glomerular filtration rates fall. Clustering of nephropathy in families suggests that there may be a genetic predisposition to nephropathy and hypertension in some individuals with type 1 diabetes.

Hypertension in people with type 2 diabetes, however, is much more common, may precede the diagnosis, and is present in between 30 and 50% at

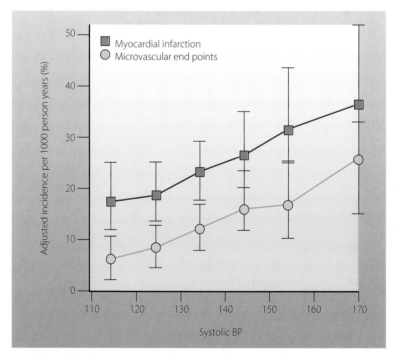

Fig. 2.7   Incidence rates (95% confidence interval) of myocardial infarction and microvascular end points by category of updated mean systolic blood pressure, adjusted for age, sex and ethnic group expressed for white men aged 50–54 years is at diagnosis and mean duration of diabetes 10 years. *BMJ* 2000; **321**: 412–19, with permission.

diagnosis. It is a major component of the metabolic syndrome that constitutes type 2 diabetes and appears to reflect insulin resistance. The effects on the cardiovascular system are more profound than similar blood pressure levels in a non-diabetic. For example, in the Multiple Risk Factor Intervention Trial Research Group (MRFIT) study, rising systolic blood pressure was associated with increasing 10 year coronary heart disease (CHD) mortality which was 3–5 times greater in those with diabetes.

Epidemiological studies have demonstrated the continuous relationship between serum cholesterol and risk of atherosclerotic vascular disease, particularly CHD. This was confirmed by the Framingham study and, in the MRFIT study when over 300 000 men aged 35–57 years were screened, the relationship between cholesterol and death from CHD was independent of smoking and hypertension and continuous across the age range. There was also a strong relationship between CHD and cholesterol level in people with diabetes.

The lipid abnormalities associated with diabetes are both qualitative and quantitive. There are no quantitive differences between patients with type 1 diabetes and non-diabetics, though abnormalities may appear with the development of nephropathy or if glycaemic control is poor. High-density lipoprotein (HDL) levels are often in the normal range but subfractions of HDL show significant differences from the normal population. For example, HDL_2 levels have a strong negative correlation with CHD and in type 1 diabetes levels of this subfraction are low, in favour of HDL_3, which does not have the same cardioprotective properties.

In type 2 diabetes the spectrum of lipid abnormalities is broader and an essential element of the metabolic syndrome. HDL levels are low, and associated with hypertriglyceridaemia. Total and LDL-cholesterol levels are similar to non-diabetic levels, but again qualitative differences exist. LDL particles are small and dense and thought to be more atherogenic. Nevertheless, LDL levels correlate with the presence of clinical macrovascular disease in both type 1 and type 2 diabetes. Hypertriglyceridaemia as a risk factor for CHD remains controversial, but accounts for some of the other lipid changes such as low HDL and the formation of small dense LDL. There are also correlations with plasminogen activator inhibitor I (PAI-I).

Smoking is an independent risk factor for macrovascular disease and in the MRFIT study increased the 10 years risk of dying from CHD by 2.4 times in non-diabetics (from 10.1 to 23.9 per 1000) and by 1.6 times in those with diabetes (from 44.5 to 68.7 per 1000). Smoking has also been implicated in the progression of microvascular and other diabetic complications including retinopathy, nephropathy and necrobiosis lipoidica. Analysis of the MRFIT data suggested that stopping smoking was one of the most effective interventions at reducing mortality from macrovascular disease.

ETHNICITY

There appear to be definite ethnic variations in the prevalence of complications of type 2 diabetes. Compared to the WESDR population of non-Hispanic whites, retinopathy is much more common in the Pima Indians of Arizona and the Mexican-Americans in San Antonio, Texas. Nephropathy is more common in indigenous peoples such as the Maori in New Zealand (**Fig. 2.8**) and south Asians. On the other hand, CHD is less frequent in the Pima Indians with type 2 diabetes than many non-diabetic white populations in the USA.

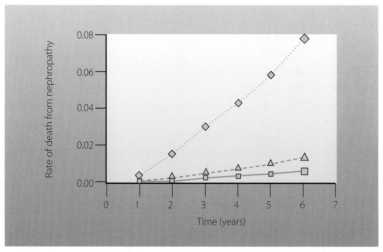

Fig. 2.8 Risk of recorded death with nephropathy by Cox's proportional hazards regression model after accounting for age, sex, and source of patient. Shown are Europeans with type 2 diabetes (□): Maori with type 2 diabetes (◇): and Pacific Islands people with type 2 diabetes (△).

CONCLUSION

Risk factors for the micro- and macrovascular complications of diabetes are similar in both type 1 and type 2 diabetes but significant differences exist in the prevalence and role of hypertension and hyperlipidaemia. Duration of diabetes is significantly correlated with complications in type 1 diabetes. An essential part of diabetes care is an annual structured risk assessment so that individual management plans can be developed to target these increased risks.

FURTHER READING

Kannel WB, McGee DL. Diabetes and glucose tolerance as risk factors for cardiovascular disease: The Framingham Study. *Diabetes Care* 1979; **2**: 120–6.

Stamler J, Vaccaro O, Neaton JD, Wentworth D. for the Multiple Risk Factor Intervention Trial Research Group. Diabetes, other risk factors and 12 years cardiovascular mortality for men screened in the Multiple Risk Factor Intervention Trial. *Diabetes Care* 1993; **16**: 434–44.

Yudkin JS. How can we best prolong life? Benefits of coronary risk factor reduction in non-diabetic and diabetic subjects. *BMJ* 1993; **306**: 1313–18.

DIABETIC NEPHROPATHY

INTRODUCTION

Diabetes is now the commonest cause of end-stage renal failure (ESRF) in Europe and North America. This is mainly because of the increasing prevalence of diabetes and because people with diabetes are now accepted more readily onto renal replacement programs, having been excluded in the past. In Scandinavia and the USA, 30% of people requiring dialysis or transplantation have diabetes though there are significant variations across Europe. Between 20 and 30% of people with type 1 or type 2 diabetes will develop nephropathy but only a small percentage of type 2 diabetics will progress to ESRF, most dying of cardiovascular disease long before the need for renal dialysis. Nevertheless, the much higher prevalence of type 2 diabetes means that up to 50% of patients with diabetes requiring dialysis are from this group.

There are considerable ethnic variations in the prevalence of nephropathy, e.g. in the UK, Anglo-Asians and Afro-Caribbeans have a much higher prevalence of nephropathy. In the USA, Pima Indians with type 2 diabetes are particularly at risk, as are the Maoris in New Zealand.

CLINICAL PRESENTATION

The earliest clinical manifestation of diabetic renal disease is the finding of small quantities of albuminuria (30–300 mg/24 h or 20–200 µg/min), often within 5–10 years of diagnosis, which increases progressively over a number of years. In cross-sectional studies, microalbuminuria is present in approximately 20–30% of insulin-treated adults and 10–30% of Caucasian adults with type 2 diabetes, and there is a clear relationship with glycaemic control (**Fig. 3.1**).

The progression of nephropathy is best documented in type 1 diabetes (**Fig. 3.2**). A history of hypertension in a first-degree relative and differences in Na^+–Li^+ counter-transport suggest there is a component related to genetic predisposition. Poor glycaemic control may initiate functional changes within 1–2 years of the diagnosis of diabetes, including renal hypertrophy and hyperfiltration with an increase in renal blood flow and glomerular filtration rate (GFR). These changes are reversible and metabolically dependent. Recent studies suggest that even levels of albumin excretion rates above 10 µg/min are highly predictive of future microalbuminuria. Blood pressure rises progressively in parallel with increasing albuminuria and secondary lipid abnormalities also occur. The glomerular barrier loses its size selectivity and as macroproteinuria is reached GFR has already started to decline. Occasionally, nephrotic syndrome may result.

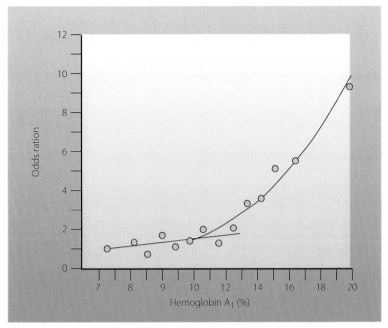

Fig. 3.1 Relation between mean haemoglobin A_1 values and the risk of microalbuminuria in patients with IDDM. *N Engl J Med* 1995; **332**: 1251–5.

The rate of decline of renal function is linear but the time to ESRF varies considerably between individuals (**Fig. 3.3**). Albuminuria is a manifestation of a generalized vasculopathy and a high proportion of nephropaths develop symptomatic coronary heart disease (CHD) in the early course of their renal disease. The associated anaemia and hypertension lead to left ventricular hypertrophy (LVH) and heart failure. Death from stroke, myocardial infarction or peripheral gangrene occurs in nearly 75% of patients, either before or during renal replacement therapy, and 50% of type 1 diabetics are dead within 10 years of the onset of proteinuria.

KEY DIAGNOSTIC FEATURES

Although the diagnosis of nephropathy is based on the finding of Albustix positive albuminuria (equivalent to a urinary albumin excretion rate of more than 300 mg/day), it is important to remember that the renal disease is already well established at the stage of overt proteinuria with irreversible structural changes having occurred in the glomeruli. In type 1 diabetes,

	Normal	Incipient nephropathy	Clinical nephropathy
UAER	<20 µg/min → 1%–2% per annum	>20 <200 µg/min (increase 20% pa) → 3%–4% per annum	<200 µg/min
GFR	Stable 1% decline pa >40 years	Age related changes; more rapid loss when UAER approaches 200 µg /min or if blood pressure increases	Decline 10 ml/min/y (hypertensive), 1–4 ml/min/y (normotensive)
Blood pressure	Stable: higher in those progressing to incipient nephropathy	Initially stable, but higher than normal UAER controls Increases with increasing UAER	Most patients hypertensive (>140/85 mmHg) Increases with declining GFR
Pathology	Large kidneys Tubular hypertrophy/ hyperplasia Glomerular enlargement Normal ultrastructure GBM thickening 20 nm pa	Kidneys remain large GBM thickening 54 nm pa Mesangial expansion ~ 4% pa	Kidneys shrink GBM 2–3 times normal, stable Nodules Global glomerulosclerosis Mesangial expansion ~ 7% pa

pa = per anum; GBM = glomerular basement membrane

Fig. 3.2 Natural history of diabetic nephropathy. From *Oxford Textbook of Medicine*, 3rd edn. Oxford University Press, 1996.

patients over 12 years of age should be screened annually for microalbuminuria using the albumin/creatinine ratio (ACR) on the first morning
urine sample (**Fig. 3.4**). Type 2 patients should be routinely screened for
albuminuria and, if Albustix negative, annual screening undertaken for
microalbuminuria, particularly if a positive result would alter or intensify
their management.

Classically, the finding of Albustix positive proteinuria on more than two
occasions in a person with established diabetes (having first ruled out urinary
tract infection) is indicative of diabetic nephropathy. Hypertension is com-

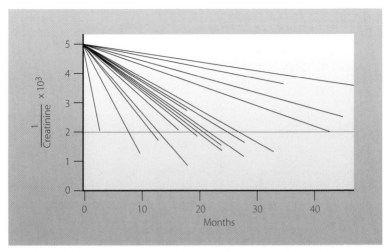

Fig. 3.3   Decline of renal function in 16 patients with nephropathy.

monly associated (**Fig. 3.5**) and the absence of retinopathy should prompt consideration of an alternative diagnosis in a patient with type 1 diabetes, but in type 2 diabetics only about 50% of those with nephropathy have associated retinopathy.

Renal ultrasound can be helpful in excluding unrelated structural abnormalities such as hydronephrosis or polycystic kidneys, but asymmetrical kidneys may be indicative of renal artery stenosis (RAS) especially in patients with peripheral vascular or aortic aneurysm disease. If renal artery Dopplers are suggestive of RAS, arteriography or CT-angiography is justified but the contrast media used for these investigations can precipitate renal failure. Adequate hydration with intravenous saline and oral treatment with acetylcysteine have been shown to substantially reduce the incidence of contrast-induced renal complications. Metformin should also be stopped 2 days before the investigation because of the risk of lactic acidosis.

Haematuria is an unusual feature in diabetic nephropathy and patients with haematuria may have coexistent renal disease unrelated to their diabetes. Renal biopsy should be considered in these patients, since it may occasionally reveal potentially treatable glomerular disease, e.g. IgA nephropathy. The morphological changes seen in the diabetic kidney, e.g. diffuse and nodular glomerulosclerosis and arteriolohyalinosis (Kimmelstiel–Wilson kidney), which may be present in over 90% of kidneys after 10 years of type 1 diabetes, are not synonymous with diabetic nephropathy. Despite these common histological changes,

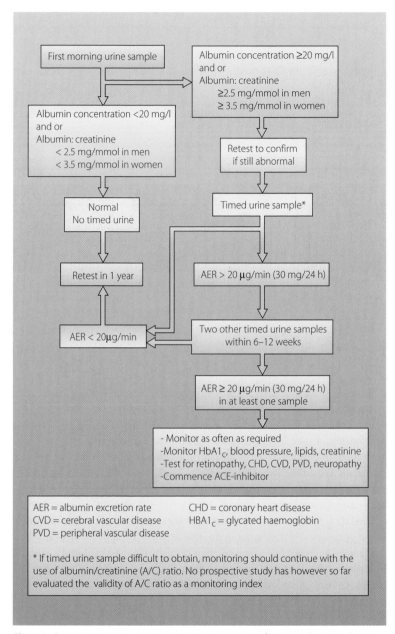

Fig. 3.4 Screening strategy and monitoring programme for microalbuminuria in type 1 diabetes.

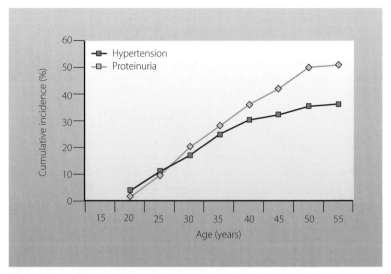

Fig. 3.5 Cumulative incidence of hypertension and persistent proteinuria in type 1 diabetes. From Williams G & Pickup JC *Handbook of Diabetes*, 2nd edn. Blackwell Science, 1997.

the clinical syndrome of nephropathy with proteinuria and declining renal function only develops in about one-third of these patients, indicating that there is a poor correlation between renal morphology and function.

EVIDENCE-BASED PRACTICE

Early detection and identification of individuals at higher risk (such as those with a family history of hypertension or a sibling with diabetes and nephropathy) should be the aim. Many of the early changes of diabetic renal disease, such as hyperfiltration and increasing albumin excretion, are readily reversible with improved glycaemic control. The Diabetes Control and Complications Trial (DCCT) showed a 39% reduction in the occurrence of microalbuminuria and a 54% reduction in albuminuria in the intensive therapy arm for both adults and adolescents with type 1 diabetes. Similarly, the United Kingdom Prospective Diabetes Study (UKPDS) showed a slowing of renal decline in the tight glycaemic control group with type 2 diabetes.

Tight control of hypertension is essential to reduce the decline in renal function. Angiotensin-converting enzyme inhibitors (ACE-Is) are indicated in type 1 patients with persistent microalbuminuria or proteinuria, irrespective of initial blood pressure, but women of childbearing age must avoid pregnancy because of potential fetal toxicity. Renoprotection by ACE-Is is probably a class effect but evidence exists for the use of captopril, enalapril and lisinopril. The sulphydril group present in captopril has antioxidant properties but whether this is advantageous in clinical practice is unproven. To achieve a target blood pressure (BP) of <130/80 for patients with nephropathy may require several antihypertensive agents and for young people under 16 years BP targets may be set even lower (to achieve a BP < 90th centile for age).

Type 2 patients with microalbuminuria or proteinuria are less likely to progress to ESRF but as with type 1 diabetes (**Fig. 3.6**) BP management is the mainstay of treatment (**Fig. 3.7**). The choice of antihypertensive drug is less important than the achieved BP but ACE-Is confer some advantages if the patient has established vascular disease, as shown in the diabetic subgroup of the Heart Outcomes Prevention Evaluation (HOPE) study (Micro-HOPE) where ramipril reduced mortality, rates of myocardial infarction and episodes of heart failure.

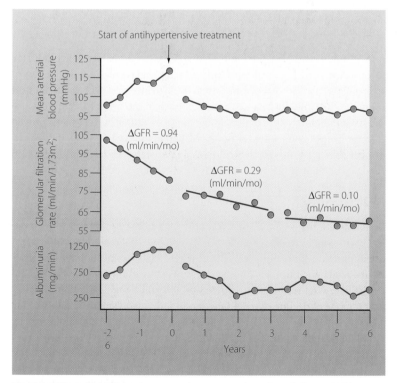

Fig. 3.6 Effect of blood pressure control on progression of renal disease in 11 patients with type 1 diabetes. *BMJ* 1987; **294**: 1443–7, with permission.

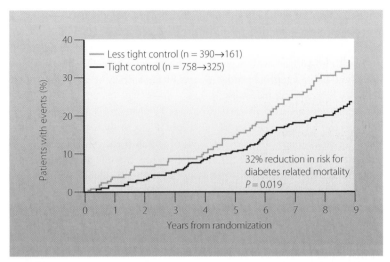

Fig. 3.7 UK Prospective Diabetes Study Group (UKPDS): blood pressure control and mortality from macrovascular disease and renal failure. *BMJ* 1998; **317**: 703–13.

Diet adjustment has a place in the management of patients with nephropathy prior to the need for renal replacement therapy, particularly with the aim of reducing vascular risk. Thus, a diet low in fat, high in antioxidants and low in salt (to reduce BP) must be balanced against potassium and phosphate intake where the serum level may be elevated. Many diabetics mistakenly eat more protein than the general population, so modest reductions can be beneficial, though low protein diets for low GFR states are not well tolerated by many patients, even though there is some evidence for their effects in slowing the deterioration.

MONITORING RENAL FUNCTION

Serum creatinine is a poor indicator of renal function, rising only after there has been a severe reduction in GFR (**Fig. 3.8**). EDTA clearance measurements are impractical for routine tracking of renal function but can be useful if 24-hour urinary creatinine clearance values are inconsistent with the clinical picture. Otherwise, reciprocal-creatinine plots against time can helpfully indicate the rate of decline of renal function in individual patients. After starting ACE-Is or AII blockers, urea and electrolytes should be monitored carefully (e.g. 1 week and 1 month after initiation) to detect hyperkalaemia or a drug-induced deterioration in renal function (usually associated with RAS).

Metformin should be avoided completely if serum creatinine is >150 µmol/l because of the potential risk of lactic acidosis. Occasional monitoring of haemoglobin, corrected calcium and fasting phosphate is indicated.

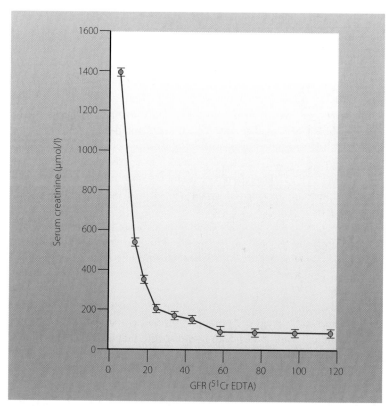

Fig. 3.8 Relationship between glomerular filtration rate (GFR) measured using chromium-51 (^{51}Cr EDTA GFR) and serum creatinine, in patients being investigated for renal disease.

Abnormal results should prompt further measurements of haematinics, especially ferritin, and indicators of bone metabolism such as alkaline phosphatase and parathyroid hormone.

Arrangements for the involvement of a nephrologist in the care of a patient with diabetic nephropathy will vary from country to country but studies in the UK have suggested that many patients are never given the opportunity of assessment by a renal physician, or else they are referred at the point of requiring dialysis. The type of patient suitable for referral to a nephrologist might be:

· patients with a serum creatinine ≥150 μmol/l;
· type 1 diabetic patients with confirmed microalbuminuria (AER > 30 μg/min);
· younger patients with overt diabetic nephropathy (dipstick positive proteinuria) but a normal serum creatinine;

- nephropaths with resistant hypertension;
- patients with asymmetrical kidneys on ultrasound or renal artery Dopplers suggestive of RAS;
- patients with overt nephropathy but atypical features such as haematuria, absence of retinopathy, or nephrotic levels of proteinuria (>3 g/24 h).

Patients with diabetic nephropathy often become symptomatic at lower serum creatinine levels than non-diabetics and thus require dialysis earlier. Choosing between haemodialysis and continuous ambulatory peritoneal dialysis (CAPD) will depend on a variety of factors including patient choice but difficulties of vascular access and problems such as coexisting autonomic neuropathy makes CAPD the preferred choice for the majority of patients. Visually impaired patients can manage CAPD surprisingly well, but they may not detect their own foot ulcers.

Symptomatic autonomic neuropathy is very much more common in diabetic nephropaths. Postural hypotension and impotence add to the concerns of the patient but one of the most distressing symptoms is gustatory sweating, which may be intolerable and is effectively untreatable. Gastroparesis is fortunately rare. All of these patients will have other diabetic complications such as retinopathy and ischaemic or neuropathic feet which need regular inspection to detect and prevent deterioration. Anaemia may respond to iron infusion but there is some evidence in non-diabetics that erythropoietin (EPO) given predialysis may slow the progression of renal deterioration (**Fig. 3.9**).

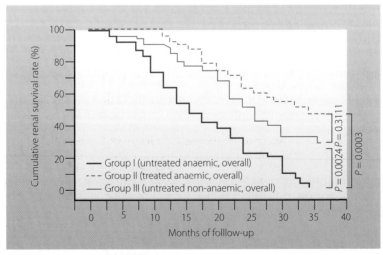

Fig. 3.9 Reversal of anaemia by erythropoietin can retard progression of chronic renal failure. *Nephron* 1997; **77**: 176–85.

CURRENT ISSUES

* Angiotensin receptor antagonists (ARAs) achieve similar reductions in BP and proteinuria as ACE-Is but the recent CALM study demonstrated that combination therapy with lisinopril 20 mg once daily and Candesartan 16 mg daily may produce superior falls in systolic and diastolic BP in comparison to either agent alone (–25/16 vs. –16/10 mmHg) in type 2 diabetics. Nevertheless, ARAs should be reserved as an alternative to ACE-Is for patients intolerant of ACE-Is (e.g. cough). As yet, there is none of the long-term data that exists for ACE-Is suggesting a specific renoprotective effect of ARAs over and above their effect on BP. They have the same renal side-effects as ACE-Is such as hyperkalaemia and must be avoided in RAS.

* Only careful attention to the cluster of vascular risk factors will begin to reduce the high mortality from CHD in these patients. Coronary risk prediction charts, e.g. those based on the Framingham data, will probably underestimate the CHD risk and should not be used in this population unless modified to adjust for proteinuria. There is good evidence to suggest that patients with nephropathy should be treated as for secondary prevention, i.e. assume they have established vascular disease and treat them at lower thresholds with statins and aspirin (once BP is controlled). There is also some evidence that statins may reduce proteinuria and have ancillary anti-inflammatory effects in the kidney.

FURTHER READING

Borch-Johnson K, Norgaard K, Homnel E *et al*. Is diabetic nephropathy an inherited complication? *Kidney Int* 1992; **41**: 719–22.

Lewis EJ, Hunsicker LG, Bain RP, Rhode RD for the Collaborative Study Group. The effects of angiotensin-converting enzyme inhibition on diabetic nephropathy. *N Engl J Med* 1993; **329**: 1456–62.

Parving HH, Anderson AR, Smidt UM, Hommel E, Mathiesen ER, Svendsen PA. Effect of antihypertensive treatment on kidney function in diabetic nephropathy. *BMJ* 1987; **294**: 1443–7.

Viberti GC, Jarrett RJ, Mahmud U, Hill RD, Argyropoulos A, Keen H. Microalbuminuria as a predictor of clinical nephropathy in insulin-dependent diabetes mellitus. *Lancet* 1982; **i**: 1430–2.

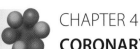

CHAPTER 4

Adrian R. Scott MD, FRCP

CORONARY HEART DISEASE AND DIABETES

INTRODUCTION

Traditionally, diabetic vascular complications are divided into microvascular and macrovascular. The uniqueness of diabetic retinopathy, and to a lesser extent nephropathy, has led to microvascular disease sometimes overshadowing the more common and life-threatening coronary and cerebrovascular events. The fascination of doctors with unusual patterns of small vessel disease has meant that for many decades the true impact of vascular disease in people with diabetes has received less attention than it deserves. Both types of diabetes are associated with a many-fold increase in the risk of macrovascular disease, particularly coronary heart disease (CHD), stroke (CVA) and peripheral vascular disease (PVD) leading to gangrene and lower limb amputation. In type 1 diabetes this is strongly associated with nephropathy but many would now consider type 2 diabetes as a cardiovascular disease *per se* since hyperglycaemia is only one element of a syndrome characterized by insulin resistance, central obesity, hypertension and hyperlipidaemia, all of which contribute to atherogenesis.

EPIDEMIOLOGY OF CHD IN DIABETES

In type 1 diabetes the risk of a vascular event increases with duration of diabetes and the presence of nephropathy. Many older studies failed to distinguish between the two major types of diabetes but the recent British Diabetic Association (BDA) cohort study followed insulin-treated patients diagnosed before the age of 30 years and found an excess of deaths at all ages. Vascular disease was implicated from the 3rd decade onwards (**Fig. 4.1**). With type 2 diabetes the increased risk of CHD is present from diagnosis and one cohort study found a history of myocardial infarction (MI) in 16.5% of males and 9.7% of females at the time of diagnosis of diabetes. During a 10-years' follow-up the age–adjusted incidence of first MI was 1.5-fold higher in diabetic men and up to 8.1-fold higher in diabetic women compared to age-matched non-diabetics. In the Framingham study, 3000 non-diabetic women were followed for 24 years and no episode of MI prior to the menopause was documented. In diabetic women before the menopause, however, the morbidity and mortality from atherosclerotic events was equal to or greater than diabetic men.

These differences in atherosclerosis between diabetics and non-diabetics are common across the world but significant differences also exist in the incidence of CHD events in diabetics from one country to another. This suggests that the risk of CHD can be modified and that environmental factors probably have a role. For example, a Central American with diabetes has less

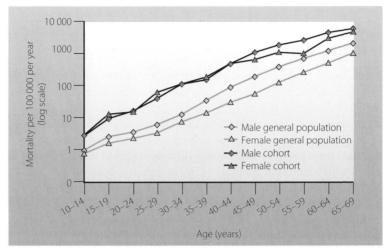

Fig. 4.1   BDA Cohort Study (1972–93): Cardiovascular disease mortality rates in insulin-treated diabetes diagnosed under age 30. *Diabetic Medicine* 1999; **16**: 466–71.

coronary atherosclerosis than a North American without diabetes. The incidence of CHD and PVD in the Japanese is very low and this is usually attributed to a diet high in carbohydrate, rich in fish and low in fat. Macrovascular complications among Japanese diabetics is one-fifth as common as among Caucasian diabetics. Hawaiian Japanese diabetics, however, have an equivalent cardiovascular mortality as Caucasian diabetics suggesting that these differences are modifiable.

AETIOLOGY

Genetics and environment contribute to the cluster of CHD risk factors associated with diabetes but fetal nutrition would also appear to have a role since small-for-dates babies are more likely to have CHD and/or type 2 diabetes in middle-age than normal birth weight babies, particularly if they also become obese (so exacerbating the hyperinsulinaemia/insulin resistance). CHD in people with diabetes is associated with the usual risk factors such as hypertension, smoking, obesity, elevated LDL-cholesterol, low HDL-cholesterol and renal disease, many of which are more common than amongst non-diabetics. The interactions are complex, however, and the Multiple Risk Factor Intervention Trial (MRFIT) study which followed over 300 000 men for 7 years found that hypertension and hyperlipidaemia had a greater impact in the diabetic subgroup (**Fig. 4.2**). Diabetic men with a cholesterol of >7.3 mmol/l were nearly six times as likely to develop CHD over the period of follow-up than

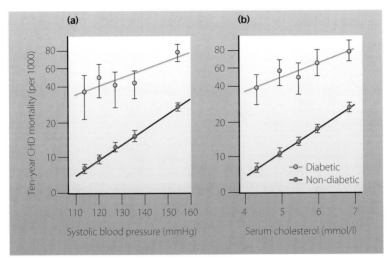

Fig. 4.2 Multiple Risk Factor Intervention Trial. Effects of systolic blood pressure (a) and serum cholesterol concentration (b) on 10-year mortality from coronary heart disease (CHD) in 342 815 non-diabetic and 5163 diabetic subjects aged 35–57 years who initially had not suffered a myocardial infarction. From Williams G & Pickup JC *Handbook of Diabetes,* 2nd edn. Blackwell Science, 1997.

diabetic men with a cholesterol level <5.5 mmol/l. Thirty per cent of smokers were dead at the end of the 7-year period.

Diabetics also have metabolic abnormalities which encourage thrombosis and discourage fibrinolysis. Thus fibrinogen, von Willebrand factor, plasminogen activator inhibitor-1 (PAI-1) and plasma viscosity are all elevated and platelet function is abnormal.

PROGNOSIS

In-hospital and 1-year mortality has been shown to be between two- and fourfold greater amongst people with diabetes, especially women. All-cause mortality in men and women aged 61–75 years admitted to hospital with an acute MI in Southern Derbyshire, UK, confirmed this pattern, with the largest number of deaths occurring within the first month (**Fig. 4.3**). The reasons for this are not clear but sudden death, heart failure and reinfarction are all more common in diabetic patients following MI. There is no evidence that infarct size is greater but underlying coronary artery atherosclerosis is more severe and there is some evidence of a cardiomyopathy associated with diabetes which could predispose to a worse outcome post-MI. A low admission blood pressure or high blood glucose level is associated with subsequent increased mortality.

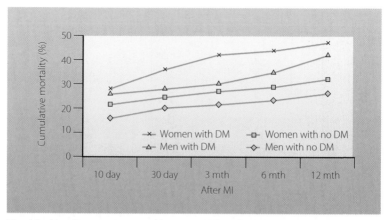

Fig. 4.3 Mortality rates in men and women with and without diabetes aged 61–75 years in Southern Derbyshire between 1995 and 1998 (unpublished data).

ASSESSING VASCULAR RISK IN PEOPLE WITH DIABETES

Stratification of risk is helpful in prioritizing care: this ensures that those with the highest risk are treated with some urgency; targets resources according to need and does not put low risk individuals at unnecessary disadvantage from long-term potential drug side-effects. All coronary risk prediction charts are based on the same Framingham data which takes into account age, gender, smoking and diabetes status, systolic blood pressure, and total cholesterol/HDL ratio. The presence or absence of left ventricular hypertrophy (LVH) and adjustment for microalbuminuria status can be included in the Framingham equations and results in an estimate of risk of a cardiovascular event (fatal or non-fatal) over a 10-year period. They are for primary prevention only, with patients categorized as high risk predicted to have over a 30% chance of an event over 10 years. To put this in context, a person with established vascular disease has a more than 40% risk over 10 years.

The original Framingham cohort was largely White and contained only a relatively small number of patients with diabetes. Thus, coronary risk prediction charts should be used with caution as they will tend to underestimate CHD risk in some ethnic groups, e.g. British Asians, patients with nephropathy and where there is a family history of premature vascular disease suggestive of a primary hyperlipidaemia.

Haffner and colleagues published evidence that the risk of death in patients with type 2 diabetes (but no prior MI) was similar to that of a non-

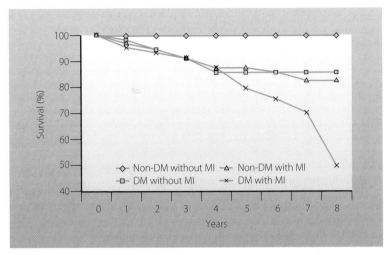

Fig. 4.4   Probability of death in 1059 subjects with type 2 diabetes and 1378 non-diabetic subjects with and without prior MI. *N Engl J Med* 1998; **339:** 229–34.

diabetics with a past history of MI (**Fig. 4.4**), suggesting that in terms of secondary prevention patients with diabetes could be considered as having the same risk of an event as someone with established vascular disease. Despite such a high risk, screening for asymptomatic CHD remains controversial. A positive exercise test in this group has a low predictive value for significant CHD on angiography. The high prevalence of hypertension (and therefore increased left ventricular mass) can give abnormal ST-segment responses to exercise as well as false positive nuclear myocardial perfusion scanning.

EVIDENCE-BASED PRACTICE

The acute management of MI in a patient with diabetes is exactly the same as for a person without diabetes, except that all diabetics (and patients with unknown diabetes status but an admission serum glucose >11 mmol/l) should receive a glucose and insulin infusion (so-called DIGAMI regimen) to maintain BG within the normal range for at least 24 hours. In the original Swedish DIGAMI studies using this i.v. regimen, patients were subsequently treated with a basal-bolus subcutaneous insulin regimen for at least 3 months and this was associated with a 29% reduction in mortality. The group which appeared to benefit most were the lower risk, younger patients on diet alone prior to the MI. Current evidence cannot distinguish between the benefits of early glucose and insulin i.v. infusion vs. the benefits attributable to post-discharge subcutaneous insulin therapy in accounting for the overall reduction in mortality, but a further DIGAMI trial (DIGAMI2) is in progress.

Effective interventions frequently show greatest benefits in the higher-risk patients and thrombolysis, beta-blockers and statins all demonstrate significantly larger absolute reductions in morbidity and mortality in the diabetic subgroups. For example, meta-analyses of beta-blocker trials show a 35% reduction in mortality when given at the time of the MI (orally or i.v.) in diabetics compared to a 13% reduction in non-diabetics. When given as secondary prevention post-MI, the corresponding results are –48% and –33%, respectively.

A similar pattern was seen with statins post-MI, e.g. in the Cholesterol and Recurrent Events (CARE) study using pravastatin 40 mg and in the Scandanavian Simvastatin Survival Study (4S) which used 20–40 mg simvastatin (**Fig. 4.5**). Reductions in mortality were greater in the diabetic subgroups, as were the reductions in duration and number of hospital admissions in the statin-treated group.

Angiotensin-converting enzyme inhibitors (ACE-Is) given post-MI reduce mortality by 22% in patients with a left ventricular ejection fraction of <40%. The Studies of Left Ventricular Dysfunction (SOLVD) demonstrated similar

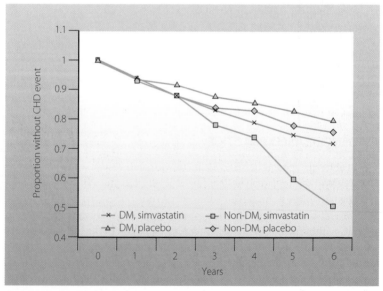

Fig. 4.5 Effects of simvastatin 20–40 mg on fatal and non-fatal cardiovascular events in diabetics and non-diabetics with known CHD: Scandanavian Simvastatin Survival Study (4S).

benefits in diabetics. The metanalysis performed by the ACE-Inhibitor Myocardial Infarction collaborative group of ACE-I therapy started on the day of MI and continued for 4–6 weeks showed that five deaths were prevented per 1000 treated patients and there was a reduced risk of heart failure. This analysis included the CONSENSUS II trial which found a negative interaction between aspirin and i.v. enalapril (a +11% increase in mortality in the enalapril group). However, in this study hypotension and severe cardiac failure at the time of randomization were not exclusion criteria. GISSI-3, using lisinopril, showed a 44% and 27% reduction in 6-week mortality in type 1 and type 2 diabetics, respectively.

The large Heart Outcomes Prevention Evaluation (HOPE) study randomized patients with CHD but clinically normal left ventricular (LV) function to ramipril 10 mg or placebo, with or without vitamin E. The diabetic subgroup (Micro-HOPE) of 3577 patients were followed for a mean of 4.5 years and treatment with ramipril was associated with a 24% reduction in all-cause mortality, 22% reduction in rate of MI and 33% reduction in rate of stroke (**Fig. 4.6**). Vitamin E had no benefit.

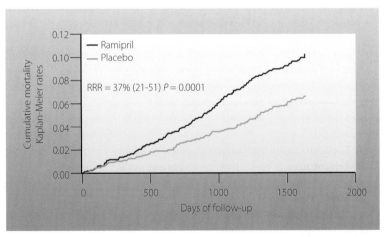

Fig. 4.6 Micro-HOPE study: Effects of ramipril or placebo on cardiovascular death in 3577 diabetics with normal left ventricular function. *Lancet* 2000; **355**: 253–9.

Does improving glycaemic control reduce cardiovascular risk?

The Diabetes Complications and Control Trail (DCCT) of conventional vs. intensive glycaemic control in type 1 diabetes was under-powered to answer this question as the cohorts were relatively young and therefore the number of events was low. There was a trend towards a reduction in cardiovascular events in the intensively treated group. The UK Prospective Diabetes Study (UKPDS) also had a non-significant (16%) reduction in fatal and non-fatal MIs in the intensively treated group after 15 years. Again, this may be because of the relatively low event rate in a group of patients who were recruited at diagnosis, were relatively young and the trial had as exclusion criteria diagnoses such as severe peripheral vascular disease and existing CHD. The previous fears raised by the University Group Diabetes Program (UGDP) in the 1970s that sulphonylureas were associated with increased cardiovascular mortality, were not realized and there appeared to be no difference between insulin and sulphonylureas in this regard. Metformin, however, used as monotherapy in the obese patient, was associated with a significant reduction in cardiovascular deaths compared to insulin or sulphonylureas. There is no long-term data on thiazolidenedione derivatives or the newer sulphonylureas.

Anti-platelet therapy

There have been no specific trials of aspirin in acute MI in people with diabetes but secondary prevention studies demonstrate a 25% reduction in cardiovascular events and 15% reduction in mortality with apparently similar results in people with diabetes. The optimal dose of aspirin remains uncertain but lower doses are associated with fewer haemorrhagic complications. Evidence of benefit of aspirin in diabetics for primary prevention must be extrapolated from trials in non-diabetics (mostly male) which suggested that there is a reduction in non-fatal cardiovascular and cerebrovascular events, that 75 mg is probably as effective as 500 mg and is not associated with an increased risk of cerebral haemorrhage in patients with controlled hypertension. There was a non-significant reduction in fatal and non-fatal MI in the Early Treatment of Diabetic Retinopathy Study using 325 mg aspirin.

Lipid-lowering therapy

Statins will reduce mortality, the need for revascularization and cardiovascular and cerebrovascular events, but the optimum dose and lipid targets remain uncertain. The British and Europeans recommend achieving a total cholesterol <5 mmol/l, and LDL <3 mmol/l, whilst the American Diabetes Association suggests an LDL target <2.6 mmol/l, HDL >1.15 mmol/l and triglycerides <2.3 mmol/l. Improved glycaemic control will enhance the lipid profile, though glitazones (more so rosiglitazone) cause a 12% increase in LDL (compensated in part by an increase in HDL). Fibrates have little effect on LDL but increase HDL and lower triglycerides. Only gemfibrozil has been shown to reduce cardiovascular mortality—which in the VA-HIT study resulted in a 22% reduction in CHD deaths or non-fatal MIs. This study included 25% diabetics and so for patients intolerant of statins, gemfibrozil 600 mg twice daily is a suitable alternative.

People with diabetes may not always be suitable for revascularization procedures as their atherosclerotic disease is often severe and widespread. Long-term survival following coronary artery bypass grafting (CABG) is less good in diabetics. The Bypass Angioplasty Revascularization Investigation (BARI) trial suggested that outcomes from angioplasty were inferior to CABG in diabetics, though whether angioplasty combined with stenting gives superior results remains to be seen.

FURTHER READING

Hales CN, Barker DJP, Clark PMS *et al*. Fetal and infant growth and impaired glucose tolerance at age 64. *BMJ* 1991; **303**: 1019–22.

Kannel WB, Mc Gee DL. Diabetes and glucose tolerance as risk factors for cardiovascular disease: the Framingham Study. *Diabetes Care* 1997; **2**: 120–6.

Laing SP, Swerdlow AJ, Slater SD. *et al*. The British Diabetic Association Cohort Study, I: all-cause mortality in patients with insulin-treated diabetes mellitus. *Diabet Med* 1999; **16**: 459–65.

Malmberg K, Ryden L, Efendic S *et al*. on behalf of DIGAMI Study Group. A randomised trial of insulin-glucose infusion followed by subcutaneous insulin treatment in diabetic patients with acute MI. (Oigami Study): effects on mortality at 1 years. *J Am Coll Cardiology* 1995; **26**: 57–65.

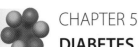

INTRODUCTION

The great disabler of all the macrovascular complications—stroke—is, as one might expect, more frequent in people with diabetes and the outcome worse than in non-diabetics. The prevalence of cerebral infarcts, especially lacunar infarcts, is increased but the prevalence of subarachnoid haemorrhage, cerebral haemorrhage, and transient ischaemic attacks are decreased, despite hypertension being so common in the diabetic patient. The presence of diabetic nephropathy and coronary and peripheral vascular disease are risk factors for stroke in the diabetic patient. Afro-Caribbeans and Afro-Americans with diabetes are particularly at risk.

A higher prevalence of stroke is found in the patient with both diagnosed and undiagnosed diabetes and glucose intolerance and, as with myocardial infarction (MI), most studies show that individuals with admission serum glucose >6.6 mmol/l have a higher morbidity and mortality.

EPIDEMIOLOGY

A number of large studies have confirmed the higher prevalence of stroke in the diabetic population. In the Framingham study, the fourfold excess in male diabetics occurred in the 5th and 6th decades, whereas in females with diabetes the excess was a decade later. Most studies (usually of hospitalized patients) suggest a relative risk of stroke 2–3 times non-diabetics, though the Swedish Gothenburg study put this excess as high as sixfold in men and 13-fold in women. Most studies have not distinguished between insulin requiring and non-insulin requiring diabetes, but for type 1 the excess may not be so great as with type 2. Certainly it is not as common as cardiovascular disease—Dekert's long-term mortality study (1976) of people with diabetes diagnosed before age 30 and followed up for more than 40 years showed a 10% incidence and 7% mortality from stroke. A similar UK study of diabetics dying before their 50th birthday found a similar mortality from stroke compared to 41% from coronary heart disease (CHD) and 19% from nephropathy.

Diabetes mellitus is associated with higher mortality, worse functional outcome, more severe disability after stroke and a higher frequency of recurrent stroke. Short- and long-term mortality is increased and in one carefully matched Finnish study, 5-year mortality was 60% in the non-diabetic controls with stroke compared to 80% in those with diabetes.

AETIOLOGY

Cerebral blood flow disturbances, impaired cerebrovascular reactivity, and damage to large and small extra- and intracranial cerebral vessels have been found in humans and animals with diabetes. Autopsy studies suggest that diabetic patients are susceptible to cerebral small-artery disease and lacunar infarction. These strokes result from vascular occlusion of small arteries at the base of the brain resulting in small deep arterial infarcts usually less than 15 mm in diameter and typically occur in hypertension and diabetes. Embolism from large vessel atheroma and heart (particularly post-infarct) is also more common. In one prospective study, carotid stenoses >50% were present in 8.2% of diabetics compared with 0.7% of age-matched controls but only 28% of diabetics with an ischaemic cerebral event had a significant carotid stenosis suggesting that smaller vessel disease is more important. The precipitant for the occlusion is not clear but appears to be linked to excessive glycation and oxidation, endothelial dysfunction, increased platelet aggregation, impaired fibrinolysis and insulin resistance. Cerebrovascular blood flow has been shown to be abnormal in people with diabetes, both of auto-regulation and in response to vasodilators such as CO_2. Endothelial dysfunction with failure to vasodilate in response to nitric oxide has been postulated; autonomic neuropathy may also be a factor.

Blood glucose on admission correlates both with survival and degree of recovery. Several studies have demonstrated a worse outcome with a presenting blood glucose >6.6 mmol/l. Whether hyperglycaemia adversely affects stroke outcome or primarily reflects stroke severity is not clear—animals studies of acute hyperglycaemia prior to cerebral ischaemia show more severe histological damage and a worse outcome but there is no evidence in humans that infarct size is larger. Hyperglycaemia might theoretically worsen stroke damage in a number of ways: the local hypoxia induced by acute cerebral ischaemia results in glucose being metabolized anaerobically causing lactic acid to accumulate. The resultant local acidosis damages vascular, glial and neuronal tissue. In addition, ischaemia causes accumulation of the neurotransmitters, glutamate and aspartate in the extracellular tissues. Usually these neurotransmitters cause stimulation of a nerve at a post-receptor site and depolarization. When accumulation occurs hyperstimulation occurs, followed by neuronal death, though glial and vascular tissue are spared. This neural toxicity may result from an increase in intracellular calcium following neuronal hyperstimulation.

CLINICAL PRESENTATION

Strokes are common and the lack of challenging interventions has often meant that these patients are not always adequately assessed and hence receive suboptimal care. Not all acute neurological events are strokes and consideration must be given to the underlying cause—classically, hypoglycaemia may present with altered consciousness but also with focal neurology and if missed, permanent neurological sequelae may result. There are also reports in the literature of focal fits and neurological signs in association with hyperglycaemia but these preceded modern scanning technology so may have represented small strokes or transient ischaemic attacks (TIAs). However, it is important not to overlook the diagnosis of non-ketotic hyperosmolar states (HONK) as the dehydration and elevated viscosity may have led to arterial occlusion causing stroke, MI, or even peripheral gangrene. Silent ischaemia is relatively common and patients may present with a stroke and uncontrolled diabetes as a complication of an earlier painless MI.

EVIDENCE-BASED PRACTICE

The reality is that acute stroke management in the person with diabetes is based on extrapolation of the data from non-diabetics as there are, as yet, no prospective studies of stroke management in diabetics. However, there is one proviso: these are high risk patients with a multisystem disorder, whom as a group do badly, both in terms of survival and rehabilitation. Early interventions must be undertaken promptly as any delay is not likely to improve prognosis.

The role of thrombolysis of acute stroke remains controversial but a systematic review of 12 controlled trials involving 3435 patients assessed the use of intravenous thrombolytic therapy (with a number of agents) started within 6 hours of the onset of symptoms of ischaemic stroke. Thrombolysis reduced the proportion of patients who died or remained dependent on others at the end of trial follow-up, up to 6 months later (61.5% vs. 68% of control patients not given thrombolysis). Results were more impressive if treatment was started within 3 hours (56.6% vs. 70.7%). Alteplase seemed superior to streptokinase but overall there was an increased risk of symptomatic intracranial haemorrhage (9.6% vs. 2.6%). Overall, the risk of dying within 2 weeks was increased in those receiving thrombolytic therapy (20.9% vs. 11.9%) despite the improvement in the composite end-point of death or dependency. Whether people with diabetes benefit similarly from thrombolysis is not known. Use of anticoagulant therapy with unfractionated or low-molecular weight heparin for acute ischaemic stroke is associated with an increase in haemorrhagic stroke but with no positive benefit in terms of mortality or dependency.

If CT scanning is not immediately available to rule out haemorrhage, administration of aspirin (orally or rectally) should, on balance, be given sooner rather than later. With the exception of immediate post-stroke hypertension management (about which little is known but for which avoidance of treatment is recommended for at least 4 weeks), correction of other comorbidities seems logical but lacks the confirmation of randomized controlled trials. Thus, dehydration and hypoxia should be avoided, with administration of antibiotics if respiratory infection supervenes. The benefits of treatment of hyperglycaemia in this situation are unknown but as it correlates with a worse outcome, a DIGAMI-style glucose and insulin infusion to maintain near-normoglycaemia would seem to be a cheap and easily implementable solution. Heparin prophylaxis is best avoided as there appears to be an increased risk of secondary cerebral haemorrhage but prevention of deep venous thromboses (DVTs) is achievable with elasticated thromboembolic stockings.

Secondary prevention data is based entirely on general population studies with none having been conducted in people with diabetes alone. General management of vascular risk factors using targets similar to those for diabetic patients with CHD would seem logical. The dose of aspirin is uncertain and some authors have suggested that people with diabetes may need higher doses to achieve the same antiplatelet effects. The European Stroke Prevention Study showed that, in the general population, aspirin and sustained-release dipyridamole are equally effective secondary prevention in reducing the risk of stroke and/or death. Addition of dipyridamole is justified if the patient has a cerebrovascular incident whilst on aspirin as this study showed that the combination was significantly more effective than either alone.

Clopidogrel is slightly superior to aspirin at the prevention of recurrent stroke but probably not cost-effective to justify widespread use. In the Clopidogrel vs. Aspirin in Patients at Risk of Ischaemic Events (CAPRIE) study 7.2% of those treated with clopidogrel 75 mg/day had an event compared with 7.7% of patients receiving aspirin 325 mg/day. It may be more affordable if patients with true aspirin allergy are targeted or those who have gastrointestinal intolerance to aspirin but not clopidogrel. Reports of thrombotic thrombocytopenic purpura with clopidogrel are worrying but fortunately rare.

Warfarin should be substituted for antiplatelet therapy if the cause of the stroke is attributable to atrial fibrillation or other emboli from the heart. It is probably safer to wait 2 weeks after the stroke before making this change.

Primary prevention of stroke in people with diabetes is of interest because there are a number of studies where stroke prevention has been a significant secondary end-point. The UK Prospective Diabetes Study (UKPDS) of hypertension, where the target for tight blood pressure control was <150/85, showed a 44% reduction in strokes compared to the less tight blood pressure control group (target BP < 180/105).

Ramipril 10 mg daily in the diabetic subgroup of the Heart Outcomes Prevention Evaluation (HOPE) study (Micro-HOPE) reduced the number of strokes from 6.1% to 4.2% (a 33% relative risk reduction) in a cohort of patients most of whom had established CHD. The difference in blood pressure between the ramipril and placebo groups at the end of the study was only 2.5/1.0—insufficient to account for the difference in stroke rates, suggesting a different mode of vascular protection by angiotensin-converting enzyme inhibitors (ACE-Is) than simply lowering blood pressure.

In both CARE and LIPID (secondary prevention studies in patients with previous MI or angina) pravastatin 40 mg reduced the risk of fatal and non-fatal cerebrovascular accidents by 31% and 20%, respectively, the numbers with diabetes, however, were too small to analyse as a separate group.

In summary, stroke prevention in people with diabetes is about aggressive management of all vascular risk factors but with an emphasis on tight blood pressure control and use of antiplatelet therapy, ACE-Is and statins. New drugs in development offer the possibility of limiting neuronal damage at the time of the acute event.

CURRENT ISSUES

- Correction of hyperglycaemia with a glucose and insulin infusion at the time of the acute stroke is the subject of a randomized control-led trial—until this reports, the DIGAMI study of glucose and insulin infusion in acute MI provides sufficient evidence to suggest that stroke patients are likely to benefit in a similar way, and uncontrolled hyperglycaemia should not be neglected.

- The place of thrombolysis in the management of acute stroke has yet to be determined and should probably only be undertaken in the context of randomized controlled trials. Current evidence suggests it must be given within 3 hours of the onset of symptoms—a goal not deliverable in most countries.

- Neuroprotective therapy remains experimental but a number of agents are being investigated. They include clomethiazole, glycine antagonists, lubeluzole and magnesium. Such treatment, given promptly after stroke onset, aims to limit ischaemic damage by protecting damaged but potentially viable neural tissue. Animal studies have suggested a neuroprotective effect of lubelozole but in humans it has not been shown to reduce neurological disability or mortality.

FURTHER READING

Antiplatelet Trialists' Collaboration. Collaborative overview of randomised trials of antiplatelet therapy—I: Prevention of death, myocardial infarction, and stroke by prolonged platelet therapy in various categories of patients. *BMJ* 1994; **308:** 81–106.

Counsell C, Sandercock P. Anticoagulant therapy compared to control in patients with acute presumed ischaemic stroke (Cochrane Review). *The Cochrane Library*, Issue 2, 1998.

Diener HC for the European and Australian Lubelozole Ischaemic Stroke Study Group. Multinational randomised controlled trial of Lubelozole in acute ischaemic stroke. *Cerebrovasc Dis* 1998; **8**: 172–81.

Wardlaw JM, Warlow CP, Counsell C. Systematic review of evidence on thrombolytic therapy for acute ischaemic stroke. *Lancet* 1997; **350**: 607–14.

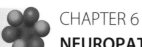

CHAPTER 6

Adrian R. Scott MD, FRCP

NEUROPATHY AND THE DIABETIC FOOT

INTRODUCTION

Foot ulceration and lower limb amputation are major causes of morbidity and disability for people with diabetes. The emotional and physical costs to the individual, as well as the huge economic cost to society, make amputation one of the most feared complications of diabetes but one that in many instances is potentially avoidable. The St Vincent declaration, now over 10 years old, set the target of reducing major lower limb amputation by 50% within 5 years. It seems unlikely that this target has actually been met, since most countries lacked the information systems needed to establish with any accuracy what were the background amputation rates, but it has highlighted the preventable nature of diabetic foot problems.

EPIDEMIOLOGY

In a lifetime, 5–10% of people with diabetes will have a foot ulcer of some degree or other. Diabetes is the commonest cause of amputation, responsible for up to 50% of non-traumatic leg amputations. Compared to the general population a person with diabetes has 15 times the risk of requiring amputation and approximately 1% will have undergone some form of amputation ranging from a single digit to major below or above knee surgery.

These patients often have multiple diabetic complications and widespread macrovascular disease with the result that coexistent disability is common making rehabilitation more complex. For this reason mobility following amputation is less satisfactory in diabetics compared to the general population. Foot ulcers commonly precede amputation, sometimes by days, weeks or months, resulting in reduced mobility and requiring a prolonged period of time off work with frequent attendances to hospital. Associated economic costs of diabetic foot disease are considerable with estimates around £13 000 000 per year in the UK. Because of coexistent complications the long-term prognosis of a person with diabetes who has had a major lower limb amputation is very poor with some estimates putting the mortality as high as 50% within 2 years of surgery.

AETIOLOGY

The Wisconsin Epidemiological Study of Diabetic Retinopathy (WESDR) was a prospective study which followed around 1200 type 1 diabetics, originally diagnosed under the age of 30, and nearly 1800 older-onset patients who were predominately type 2 (around 800 of whom were treated with insulin).

Approximately 1300 of this study population were followed up at 10 years—the main reason for the dropout was death before 10 years. The incidence of retinopathy, and progression of retinopathy, increased from the lowest to the higher quartile of $HbA1_C$. There was also a relationship between $HbA1_C$ and the incidence of nephropathy and macrovascular disease with increased risk of amputation in both younger and older groups. In the UK Prospective Diabetes Study (UKPDS) the risk of each of the microvascular and macrovascular complications of type 2 diabetes was strongly associated with hyperglycaemia as measured by $HbA1_C$. There was no evidence of a threshold and there was a threefold increase over the range of <6% to >10%.

Foot ulceration or amputation is more common in people with a long duration of diabetes (more than 10 years), especially males with poor glycaemic control, and macrovascular, retinal or renal complications are often present. Risk factors for foot ulceration include the following:

· peripheral neuropathy resulting in loss of protective sensation;
· pre-existing (often non-diabetes related) foot deformity such as hallux valgus as well as altered bio-mechanics as a result of neuropathy lead to areas of increased pressure and callus formation;
· peripheral vascular disease (PVD); and
· previous foot ulceration or amputation of the other leg.

The elderly are particularly at risk because of their frequent inability to reach or inspect their feet which is compounded often by poor vision. Lack of diabetes education has also been associated with an increased risk of foot ulceration.

A number of these risk factors often cluster together in the same person. Tissue breakdown and ulceration may occur as the result of abnormal pressure loading on the sole of the foot which invariably leads to callus formation—an important component in the lead up to ulceration. Unchecked, the callus builds up, increasing pressure loading and ulceration may occur beneath the callus where haemorrhage or necrosis begins and ultimately breaks through the skin surface. Alteration in the architecture of the foot leads to changes in shape, which normal footwear cannot accommodate and ulceration may occur at these points of excessive contact. Once the integrity of the skin has been broken, infection may swiftly follow particularly with a defective microcirculation that will impair oxygen and nutrient transport. Deeper tissues rapidly become involved and osteomyelitis is a common finding.

Ulcers may be predominantly neuropathic or ischaemic, but frequently are a combination of both. Most studies have shown that significant neuropathy is present in over 80% of patients with foot ulceration. Neuropathy has sensory, motor and autonomic components, all of which probably contribute to foot ulceration. Sensory modalities are lost at different rates and temperature perception is one of the first to be affected. Vibration perception threshold increases and is associated with risk of foot ulceration but is a feature of advancing age as well as of diabetic neuropathy. Tuning forks are inconsistent but a biothesiometer produces a vibration which can be increased in frequency and a perception threshold determined. Thresholds have been determined which predisposed to foot ulceration. Sensation to light touch and deep pressure are lost progressively.

Motor neuropathy particularly affects the intrinsic muscles of the foot with the result that the unaffected long extensors cause clawing of the toes. The plantar fascia may rupture. Subluxation of the metatarsal heads occurs and the transverse arch of the foot is lost (**Fig. 6.1**). Both the dorsum of the toes and the head of the metatarsals now become vulnerable to ulceration. The altered bio-mechanics of the diabetic neuropathic foot along with any pre-existing non-diabetic deformity, such as hallux valgus, greatly increases the risk of ulceration.

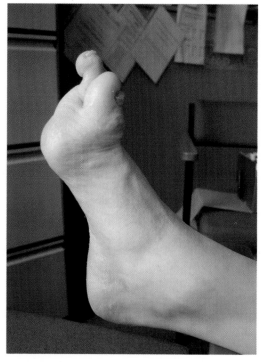

Fig. 6.1 Neuropathic foot with deformity due to subluxation of meta-tarsal heads.

CLINICAL PRESENTATION

Systems of care must be able to identify patients with at-risk feet and give them the appropriate education, nail and foot care and where appropriate, protective footwear, all of which have been shown to reduce the risk of ulceration and amputation. A number of scoring systems and assessment tools have been developed (**Fig. 6.2**); these can be used for assigning a level of risk to the individual's foot. This alerts both patient and health professional, though in itself is insufficient as the patient must be given very clear instructions on what steps to take in the event, say, of developing a foot ulcer. Sometimes the diagnosis of diabetes is made when the person presents with a foot ulcer. For reasons that are not clear these are often men and coexistent retinopathy is commonly present. In the majority, however, there is a history of 'mild type 2 diabetes' where the development of foot deformity, neuropathy and perhaps peripheral vascular disease has gone largely unnoticed. The patient presents wearing quite inappropriate shoes and the ulcer will have developed either under an area of callus or over an area of excessive contact such as the tip or dorsum aspect of claw toes, or the medial aspect of the great toe or lateral border of the 5th toe. There is little depth of tissue to protect the underlying interphalangeal joint and infection rapidly invades joint and bone. An obvious cellulitis (**Fig. 6.3**) may occur which spreads over the foot and may be accompanied by systemic symptoms such as rigors. Often, however, the infection is less obvious and these toes have a typical 'sausage' appearance—swollen throughout their length, somewhat discoloured but not grossly cellulitic. On passive movement the toe feels floppy and this combination of signs indicates underlying osteomyelitis. The neuropathic foot can look deceivingly healthy because of its warmth and bounding foot pulses but a simple means for assessing protective sensation uses a nylon monofilament, which delivers a standard pressure. The filament bends as it delivers a particular pressure and a 10-g monofilament has been shown to identify patients at risk of foot ulceration. There is often a marked absence of sensation often to the ankle or even higher.

Peripheral vascular disease is very common and may be asymptomatic and coexist with the neuropathy. When severe the appearance of the ischaemic foot is quite different from one where neuropathy predominates. The subcutaneous fat is absent, small muscles are wasted, the skin hairless. On dependency the toes appear red—rapidly developing pallor on elevation and if arterial input is very poor, venous guttering occurs. Often the disease is distal and a popliteal pulse remains palpable; more proximal disease offers the hope of vascular reconstruction or angioplasty but this can only be determined by

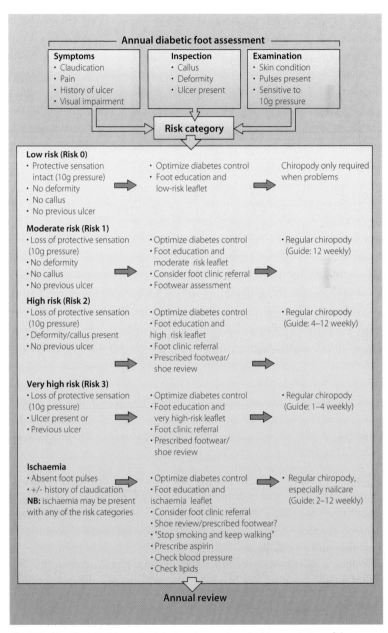

Fig. 6.2 Modified Blackburn Foot Protocol reproduced with permission of the Blackburn Diabetic Foot Team.

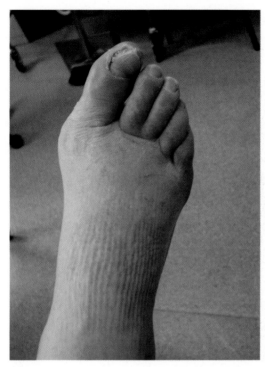

Fig. 6.3 Ischaemic foot with cellulitis great toe.

more detailed investigation either with duplex ultrasound or angiography. Measurement of ankle/brachial blood pressure ratio may be misleadingly reassuring in people with diabetes, as arteries are stiff and give falsely elevated ankle pressures.

Gross changes in the architecture of the foot, particularly at the ankle or midfoot, suggest Charcot arthropathy (**Fig. 6.4**). There may be a history of minor injury or fracture and the patient may have noticed some swelling which is usually painless. The skin over the area is hot in the absence of other signs of infection (ulceration over the deformity can make differentiation from infection very difficult).

Wagner's classification of foot ulcers is very useful for auditing care (**Table 6.1**).

EVIDENCE-BASED PRACTICE

Neither the Diabetes Control and Complications Trial (DCCT) nor UKPDS were powered to look at PVD or an amputation as an end-point—DCCT patients were young and few had macrovascular events; UKPDS patients with

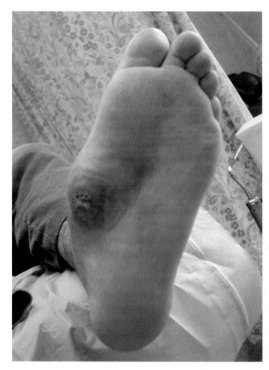

Fig. 6.4 Charcot foot showing deformity due to subluxation of talus and ulceration of overlying skin.

Wagner's classification of diabetic foot lesions

Grade 0	High-risk foot, no ulcer
Grade 1	Superficial ulcer, not clinically infected
Grade 2	Deeper ulcer, often with cellulitis; no abscess or bone infection
Grade 3	Deep ulcer with bony involvement or abscess formation
Grade 4	Localized gangrene (toe, forefoot or heel)
Grade 5	Gangrene of the whole foot

Table 6.1 Wagner's classification of diabetic foot lesions.

significant PVD at diagnosis were excluded from the study. There was no difference between the intensive and conventional treatment groups in the proportion of patients who had evidence of PVD by Doppler blood pressure or absent peripheral pulses. In the primary prevention cohort of the DCCT, intensive therapy delayed the appearance of neuropathy at 5 years by 69%. Ten per cent of the conventional treatment group developed neuropathy compared to 3% in the conventional group. Progression (as judged by clinical findings and nerve conduction studies) was reduced by 59%.

No controlled trials have been undertaken with diabetic patients to assess the effects of risk factor modification on the regression of vascular disease, however, smoking cessation is associated with improvement of symptoms in non-diabetics. Among patients with symptomatic PVD, continued smoking is associated with worsening claudication, limb-threatening ischaemia and amputation, and the need for revascularization. Patency rates are lower following revascularization in patients who continue to smoke and survival is reduced. The effects of management of hyperlipidaemia and hypertension on the progression of PVD has not been fully evaluated but an analysis of the Scandanavian Simavastatin Survival Study (4S) study showed that the incidence of 'new or worsening claudication' was significantly lower in coronary heart disease (CHD) patients treated with SImvastatin. In the Physician's Health study, low doses of aspirin resulted in a 54% reduction in the risk of peripheral arterial surgery, compared with placebo.

The greatest impact on limb preservation in the diabetic patient, however, has been the development of multidisciplinary teams, involving physician, vascular surgeon, nurse specialist, chiropodist (podiatrist) and orthotist. The realization that the neuropathic foot ulcer will heal, given appropriate antibiotic treatment of infection and relief of excess pressure, has transformed surgical practice in many countries, where the traditional approach to diabetic foot ulceration was amputation particularly if there was evidence of underlying osteomyelitis. Neuro-ischaemic and ischaemic ulceration may be more difficult to heal but the joint management approach still applies, together with aggressive revascularization, either by angioplasty or vascular reconstruction. Amputation still has a place, however, particularly where there is intractable pain or if the alternative is prolonged hospitalization with an uncertain outcome. Some patients will choose amputation knowing that life expectancy is reduced and preferring to improve their quality of life. Unfortunately, many of these patients have multiple complications, together with cardiac and renal impairment and chronic ill-health is the norm.

All feet with ulcers need radiographs though these may be normal in both early osteomyelitis and Charcot arthropathy and a repeat X-ray a few weeks later is usually necessary.

Infection is common though it is not always easy to tell if this is significant or if the deeper tissues are involved. The commonest organisms are *Staphylococcus aureus* and anaerobes. Multiple-resistant *Staphylococcus aureus* is increasingly common and will influence the choice of antibiotic. There have been no definitive randomized controlled trials and most practice has been arrived at through consensus (and anecdote). Where there is evidence of acute cellulitis, intravenous therapy is advised with broad spectrum antibiotics such as a combination of ampicillin, flucloxacillin and metronidazole, though the exact choice will depend on locally developed guidelines in the context of knowledge regarding bacterial sensitivities. The duration of intravenous therapy will depend on the clinical response but may be for a week or more. With less acute infections and where underlying osteomyelitis is suspected, a prolonged course of oral clindamycin with ciprofloxacin, or amoxycillin-clavulanate works well. Pseudo-membranous colitis was reported with clindamycin when more widely used, but in practice is rarely seen particularly if the patient is advised to discontinue therapy if diarrhoea occurs. Regular cleaning of the foot and the ulcer is essential and should be probed to localize any collections of pus or bits of bone. Surgery may be required to aid drainage or debride particularly large areas of necrotic tissue.

The choice of dressing remains to be determined as there have been few randomized trials. When infection and slough have been reduced to the minimum there is some evidence that platelet-derived growth factor may promote healing. Live-cultures of human dermal tissue (originally from neonatal foreskin) has also resulted in accelerated healing but both therapies are costly and experience with them limited.

Signs of infection in the ischaemic foot may be masked but pain is suggestive. If in doubt it is always better to treat with antibiotics because diabetic foot ulceration is clearly an emergency—infection in an ischaemic toe can rapidly lead to digital arterial thrombosis and gangrene. Prompt treatment with antibiotics is essential; the addition of aspirin, and possibly heparin, is unproven but seems logical. An urgent vascular opinion with a view to angioplasty has not been shown to reduce the incidence of amputation compared with conservative treatment but many clinicians feel that it has a place. Certainly, digital gangrene can be a disaster necessitating major lower limb amputation if distal disease is severe and not amenable to reconstruction.

Pressure-relieving removable casts can be custom-made and allow the patient to mobilize whilst still protecting the ulcer. Charcot joints can be very difficult to manage but in the acute phase where the joint is very hot and blood flow markedly increased, the consensus is to immobilize with a below-knee cast and to make the patient non-weight bearing until there are signs of less activity (usually by observing a fall in skin temperature over the affected joint). Non-steroidal anti-inflammatory drugs (NSAIDs) can be given but their role is uncertain. Intravenous pamidronate has been shown to reduce markers of bone turnover, local temperature and swelling and may have a place. The duration of casting will depend upon clinical response.

Once ulcers have healed, the next phase is to reduce the risk of this happening again. Patient education is essential and the orthotist can supply the appropriate footwear to protect against future ulceration.

CURRENT ISSUES

- Drug treatment to prevent or reverse neuropathy has been disappointing. Aldose reductase inhibitors have demonstrated little or no clinical benefit and other agents such as essential fatty acids (omega-6 and omega-3) are under investigation. Omega-6 EFAs such as gamma-linoleic acid is derived from vegetable sources such as evening-primrose oil and omega-3 EFAs from marine fish. Both are very metabolically active, improving lipid profiles, reducing platelet aggregation and acting as precursors for vasodilators such as prostanoids, leucotrienes and prostaglandins. The beneficial effects seen in animals on preservation of nerve-conduction velocity have not been so convincing in humans with diabetes but further trials are awaited.
- The impact of statins on the progression (and regression) of diabetic peripheral vascular disease has not been subject to study but the large UK Heart Protection study due to complete at the end of 2001, includes a large cohort with peripheral vascular disease and diabetes.
- Duration of antibiotic therapy and their role in 'clean' foot ulcers is uncertain—there have been no randomized controlled studies nor are any planned as far as the author is aware.

FURTHER READING

Boulton AJM, Connor H, Cavanagh PR, eds. *The Foot in Diabetes*, 2nd edn. Chichester: John Wiley and Sons, 1994.

ERECTILE DYSFUNCTION

INTRODUCTION

Diabetes may lead to sexual dysfunction in both men and women. For the purposes of this book it is not possible to consider diabetes-related sexual dysfunction in women though the causes are similar in both genders. For years the treatment of erectile dysfunction (ED) was complex, unsatisfactory and disliked by patients and/or their partners. Embarrassment lead to a conspiracy of silence: 'I won't ask if you won't say'—and this important and distressing complication was too often ignored. With the advent of oral therapies for ED and the publicity surrounding the launch of Viagra, there has been much more open discussion so that even though one-third of diabetic men will not respond to sildenafil, the dialogue has begun and other treatment avenues can be explored. This chapter looks at the aetiology of ED in people with diabetes, the importance of a correct diagnosis, followed by a look at past, present and future treatments.

Sexual function declines with age and it must be remembered that the range of normal in describing sexual activity is very wide. It is estimated that as many as 25% of men over 65 suffer from ED and in the diabetic population this is much higher—published studies vary, but quoted ranges are between 30 and 60% suffering from partial or complete ED with ejaculatory abnormalities such as retrograde ejaculation occurring in a smaller proportion.

CLINICAL PRESENTATION

The term ED is preferred to impotence as there are clearly grades of dysfunction and impotence has such negative connotations of failure. An erection insufficient for intercourse is the usual definition and the skill of the clinician is to allow the patient to acknowledge there is a problem without intimidating them with what could be seen as overly intrusive questions. Nevertheless, a clear description of the onset and type of problem is essential if the appropriate treatment is to be selected.

Intermittent or occasional erectile failure is very common and usually due to anxiety, alcohol or sexual indifference. How the partner copes with this failure can often determine future function—annoyance, anger or even ridicule will heighten anxiety on future attempts, leading to 'performance anxiety' and recurrent failure. This is perhaps the commonest cause of ED in the non-diabetic population. Diabetics are not immune to this type of failure and anxiety may be exacerbated by their awareness of ED as a complication of diabetes.

Mechanical problems such as phimosis (caused by hyperglycaemia-induced balanitis) or Peyronie's disease may be concealed in the patient's description and should be specifically asked for. Erectile dysfunction can be a manifestation of depression (as well as leading to it) so questions regarding sleep pattern, self-worth, mood, etc. are important. A loss of libido is not typical of ED due to diabetes and may suggest depression, hypogonadism or chronic ill-health. Chronic alcohol dependency as well as acute binges are other causes.

The natural history of sexual function in man is variable but changes and declines with age. Most organic causes of ED result in preserved libido but are associated with a relatively slow onset of loss of spontaneous erections, especially those present on waking. Erectile dysfunction only with their partner but not in response to auto-erotic stimuli such as masturbation strongly suggests psychogenic causes. It is essential to explore the relationship (if there is one) as dysharmony will usually cause sexual tension and could lead to ED. Attitudes of the male to sex may need to be explored, as for many, an erect penis is confirmation of their manhood and successful place in society. Sexual failure can lead to shame or anger towards their partner and the mistaken belief that sex equals penetration leads them to withdraw from all physical contact, leaving them very isolated.

AETIOLOGY

It is too simplistic to attribute impotence to autonomic neuropathy or macrovascular disease. There is a clear association with microvascular disease including retinopathy and renal disease and most patients have abnormal cardiovascular reflexes and/or peripheral neuropathy. However, the converse is not true—many patients have abnormal autonomic function but normal sexual function.

It is worth considering the mechanisms of normal erection which after the appropriate sexual stimulation, depends on relaxation of the smooth muscle of the corpus cavernosa allowing expansion of the lacunar spaces against the tunica albuginea, the mechanical compression of subtunical venules and the entrapment of blood in corpus cavernosa. This increased arterial flow into the penis is achieved by dilatation of the penile arteries. Nervous control of erection is mediated by parasympathetic fibres from the 2nd and 3rd sacral nerve roots. Sympathetic activity fibres arise mainly from the lower thoracic (T11) down to the 2nd lumbar nerve root and are mainly associated with ejaculation and detumescence. These autonomic fibres travel with somatic fibres in the pudendal nerve which comes off the sciatic nerve.

An essential part of the mechanism leading to penile erection is non-adrenergic, non-cholinergic relaxation of vascular and cavernous smooth muscle resulting in blood flow up to 100 ml/min. A number of chemical pathways are involved but the most important is the release of nitric oxide (NO) which stimulates the formation of cyclic GMP (cGMP) by guanylate cyclase (**Fig. 7.1**). Cyclic GMP relaxes smooth muscle by decreasing intracellular calcium and an erection ensues. Detumescence occurs when cGMP is broken down by phosphodiesterase type 5 (PDE 5). Prostaglandins (PG) also play a role in erection and detumescence. Other chemicals include vasoactive intestinal polypeptide (VIP), purinergic agonists, e.g. adenosine, endothelin, and neuropeptide-Y. Diabetes has effects on the neural and vascular elements of erection and penile biopsies from impotent diabetic men showed reduced number of immunoreactive nerves as well as

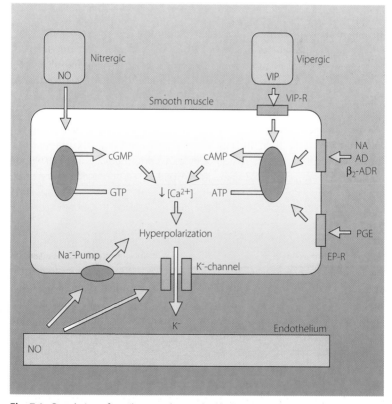

Fig. 7.1   Regulation of penile smooth muscle relaxation: cGMP, cAMP and hyperpolarization. (NA, noradrenaline; AD, adrenaline; β_2-ADR, β_2-adrenergic receptor; EP-R, prostaglandin E receptor; VIP-R, vasoactive intestinal peptide receptor; NO, nitric oxide.

VIP immunoreactivity. Diabetes causes inhibition of PG synthesis and cigarette smoking causes acute vasoconstriction of the penile arterial blood flow by inhibiting PGI_2 synthesis. Hyperlipidaemia disrupts both PG and NO synthesis at a vascular endothelial level and is frequently part of the diabetic metabolic syndrome.

KEY DIAGNOSTIC FEATURES

It is not always possible to differentiate between psychogenic and organic ED as there is often overlap, particularly in the man with diabetes. Also, it is easy to assume that all ED is a result of their diabetes which should be a diagnosis arrived at by excluding other causes (**Table 7.1**). The multiple comordidities in people with diabetes means they are frequently on drugs that may interfere with sexual function. Antihypertensives are a particular problem but unless there is a clear history associating the onset of ED with drug therapy it is usually an unrewarding task to stop one agent and try another. The UK Prospective Diabetes Study (UKPDS) showed that over one-third of patients need three or more drugs to control hypertension and ultimately the patient may have to face the difficult choice between well-controlled hypertension and erectile function. Frequently, however, the ED is a result of the diabetes and the presence of microvascular complications increases this possibility. The onset is gradual, with the patient observing a reduction in the quality of erections and spontaneous early morning erections become increasingly scarce. The sensation of ejaculation diminishes and retrograde ejaculation may occur. Libido remains normal unless depression supervenes.

Causes of erectile dysfunction
• Macrovascular disease
• Microvascular disease
• Surgical or traumatic damage to pelvic vasculature
• Neurological disorders, e.g. MS
• Spinal cord damage/disease
• Autonomic neuropathy
• Hypogonadism
• Psychogenic
• Previous priapism
• Peyronie's disease
• Drugs: antihypertensives, antidepressants, tranquillizers, anti-androgens etc.
• Chronic liver/renal disease

Table 7.1 Causes of erectile dysfunction.

EVIDENCE-BASED PRACTICE

Although the diagnosis is usually made on the history, a careful physical examination is important, particularly of the genitals looking for evidence of hypogonadism or phimosis. A few simple blood tests should be done in all patients but more sophisticated investigations such as autonomic function tests and penile vascular studies are rarely necessary outside of the research setting (**Table 7.2**). Sex hormone binding globulin may be helpful in interpreting a borderline low testosterone.

Minimum investigations in the assessment of erectile dysfunction in a patient with diabetes
• Physical examination
• Testosterone
• Prolactin
• Gonadotrophins
• Sex hormone binding globulin

Table 7.2 Minimum investigations in the assessment of erectile dysfunction in a patient with diabetes.

Involvement of the partner at an early stage should be encouraged as their cooperation is essential if treatment is to be successful. Options for treatment include, of course, no therapy and many couples may opt for this having modified their sexual lifestyle to accommodate the male partner's ED. For others, just the open discussion and the restoration of physical contact without sex is enough. The treatment options are as follows:

- Sildenafil is a selective inhibitor of PDE5—the enzyme responsible for breaking down cGMP. It therefore helps to restore natural erectile function but will only work in the presence of sexual stimulation. An overall response rate of 80% has been reported (**Fig. 7.2**) but in diabetic men up to one-third gain little benefit even with the larger dose (100 mg). It is taken about an hour before sexual activity starting with 50 mg and adjusting the dose according to response. Headache, flushing and nasal congestion have all been reported. Sildenafil may potentiate the hypotensive effects of nitrates and use in these patients is contraindicated. Early fears of sudden deaths in patients taking sildenafil have not been borne out but it must be remembered that intercourse can be very physical and in patients with a high prevalence of coronary heart disease may be potentially harmful.

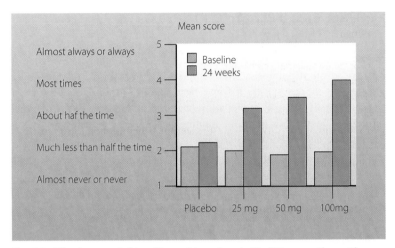

Fig. 7.2 Effectiveness of sildenafil over 24-week period in 216 men with erectile dysfunction (ED). *Br J Urology* 1996; **78**: 257–61.

- Intracavernosal injection therapy has been superseded by oral sildenafil but nevertheless remains a useful second-line therapy if sildenafil is unsuccessful or contraindicated. Unlicensed drugs include papaverine (a non-specific PDE inhibitor) which can be used alone or with phento-lamine (an alpha-blocker), and VIP. However, the only licensed product is Prostaglandin E1 (PGE_1) (alprostadil) which has an overall response rate of 70–80%. Erection occurs within 5–20˙min, it is rapidly metabolized and the incidence of priapism low, but the invasive nature of the treatment is unacceptable to many men and there is always a high drop-out rate. Pain may occur at the injection site and repeated injections into the same site has been reported to cause areas of fibrosis. Use should be limited to once a week and careful instructions given to the pa;tient to immediately report to the hospital if the erection lasts for more than 6 hours. Repeated hip movements or going for a brisk walk can cause detumesence probably by diverting blood to the legs but if priapism persists penile aspiration is required.
- Transurethral drug application using a narrow pellet of synthetic PGE1 reportedly has a success rate of 60–70%. Erection is normally achieved within 5–10˙min and lasts for up to an hour but local pain is a common problem leading to discontinuation of this form of therapy. There is a low risk of priapism.
- Vacuum constriction devices were first invented in the late 19th century to enhance penile function. However, it was not until the 1980s that they

began to be used successfully in the treatment of ED. There are three components to the device:
- a cylinder with one open end into which the penis is inserted;
- a vacuum pump (hand or battery operated); and
- a constriction ring.

Creating a vacuum in the tube causes blood to be drawn into the penis producing an erection—the ring is slipped off the cylinder onto the base of the penis to maintain rigidity. This is sufficient for penetration in the majority of patients. The ring should not be left on for more than 30 min and correct training in the use of this device is essential if successful and safe use is to be achieved. Couples complain about the lack of spontaneity with vacuum devices.

- Surgery has a very limited place in the treatment of ED but several penile prosthetic implants are available. The high cost and risk of infection limit their use.
- Penile constriction rings (as used with vacuum devices) can sometimes be helpful in those men with partial ED by increasing penile engorgement.
- Yohimbe has been the subject of a number of double blind trials with conflicting results but is not licensed for use in the UK. It has only modest effects at best.
- Transcutaneous nitroglycerine has not been confirmed to be of use in ED.
- Combination therapies may have to be used if only a partial response is seen with one treatment alone.

CURRENT ISSUES

- Phentolamine mesylate an oral alpha-adrenoceptor blocker has a faster onset of action than sildenafil. At doses of 40 mg and 80 mg about a half of those treated managed an erection sufficient for penetrative sex on 75% of attempts.
- Other oral agents under development include derivatives of yohimbine and delquamine which are centrally acting adrenoceptor antagonists.
- Oral apomorphine has recently been licensed for the treatment of ED and in a study of 854 patients (16% with diabetes) the 4 mg dose resulted in a rapid onset erection in 50% of patients. The main side-effect is nausea which generally decreases with use.

FURTHER READING

Burnet AL. Nitric oxide in the penis: physiology and pathology. *J Urol* 1997; **157**: 320–24.

Maggi M *et al.* Erectile dysfunction: from biochemical pharmacology to advances in medical therapy. *Eur J Endocrinol* 2000; **143** (2): 143–54.

Porst H. Current perspectives on intracavernosal pharmacotherapy for erectile dysfunction. *Int J Impot Res* 2000; **12** (Suppl. 4); S91-S100.

Rajfer J. Opportunities and challenges in oral therapy. *Int J Impot Res* 2000; **12** (Suppl. 4): S59-S61.

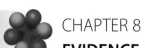

CHAPTER 8
EVIDENCE-BASED INTERVENTIONS TO PREVENT OR RETARD VASCULAR COMPLICATIONS

INTRODUCTION

It was not until very late in the 20th century that physicians began to see diabetes (particularly type 2 diabetes) as a vascular disorder and for reasons that seem unclear now, these patients were excluded (along with women) from many of the ground-breaking trials to prevent vascular complications by the treatment of hypertension, hyperlipidaemia, etc. With the exception of treatment of hyperglycaemia, there have been very few primary or secondary prevention studies that only include patients with diabetes. Much of our information on interventions that prevent or retard the vascular complications of diabetes are derived from either subgroup analyses of larger trials, or extrapolation of data from the non-diabetic population to those with diabetes. In general, however, where an intervention has been shown to reduce risk in the general population, the benefit to those with diabetes has been even greater.

A word of caution: throughout this section I have emphasized that relative risk reduction has to be seen in the context of the base-line risk and the benefits of intensive treatment, whether it be of glycaemic control, lipids or hypertension must be viewed against both the cost and potential for harm, of this approach, vs. the outcomes of a less intensive approach. This is best summed up by an analysis of the UK Prospective Diabetes Study (UKPDS) of conventional vs. intensive control of blood glucose and hypertension (**Table 8.1**). When viewed in terms of the events prevented by more intensive therapy of hyperglycaemia, one view is that the results are quite disappointing. Others would argue that these benefits were actually achieved by only a small mean difference in $HbA1_C$ (1%) and that interventions that achieve even tighter control are likely to show even greater benefits. Whilst clinicians have to try and make sense of these dilemmas, the challenge is to help people with diabetes make informed choices about their therapy—some will view a weight gain of 5 kg (the mean likely to occur with intensive insulin therapy) unacceptable if the health gain is as follows: out of 100 newly diagnosed patients, with intensified therapy (mean $HbA1_C$ 7%), 41 will develop a diabetes-related end-point (DREP) over 10 years but if glycaemic control is less tight (mean $HbA1_C$ 7.9%) 46 will develop a DREP. Unfortunately, the person opting for insulin therapy (and 5 kg weight gain) cannot assume that they will be one of the 5 out of the 100 who will benefit.

Various ways of presenting identical data on the effects of intensified vs. conventional therapy on 'any diabetes-related endpoint'		
	Intensified therapy 100 patients over 10 years median HbA1$_c$ 7%	**Conventional therapy** 100 patients over 10 years median HbA1$_c$ 7.9%
Patients with at least one endpoint		
No. of patients (%)	41 (41%)	46 (46%)
Patients without any endpoint		
No. of patients (%)	59 (59%)	54 (54%)
		Differences
Benefit of intensified vs. conventional therapy		
Decrease in patients with endpoint		
No. of patients		5
Absolute risk reduction		5%
Relative risk		11%
Increase in patients without endpoint		
No. of patients		5
Absolute increase		5%
Relative increase		9%
Lack of benefit of intensified vs. conventional therapy		
Patients with endpoint despite intensified therapy		
No. of patients		41
Absolute per cent		41%
Relative per cent (41 of 46)		89%
All patients who do not benefit		
No. of patients (%)		95 (95%)

Table 8.1 Various ways of presenting identical data on the effects of intensified vs. conventional therapy on 'any diabetes-related endpoint'.

Despite the wealth of information available to clinicians we are unable to quantify the benefit of *multiple* proven interventions against no treatment, but we can be fairly confident that both quality and quantity of life are improved in the short to medium term. What uncertainty must not do is lead to inaction or sloppy clinical practice—for example, debate over which is the most appropriate blood pressure target should not prevent a pragmatic

approach that aims to achieve a sustainable reduction in blood pressure without causing unacceptable side-effects. Similarly, prescribing the latest lipid-
lowering agent is insufficient, if an annual assessment of the foot to identify
at-risk features is omitted since this simple intervention has been demonstrated to reduce the risk of lower limb amputation.

EVIDENCE-BASED INTERVENTIONS

Macrovascular disease—Acute coronary syndromes (ACS), primary and secondary prevention of coronary heart disease

Thrombolysis/anticoagulation
Several large trials have proved the efficacy of thrombolysis for acute myocardial infarction (AMI) with a variety of agents such as streptokinase, uroki-
nase, tissue plasminogen activator (TPA) or similar. No trials have been conducted in diabetics alone. The earlier the treatment is given the better the outcome and the absolute benefit at the 5th week is 30 lives saved per 1000
patients treated before the 6th hour and 20 lives saved per 1000 patients treated between the 6th and 12th hour. The mortality benefit persists at 1 year and
beyond. The maximum reduction in mortality was achieved in those patients
treated during the first hour after the onset of symptoms. The benefit of
thrombolysis is significant regardless of age, gender, previous MI or diabetes.
In fact, although the relative risk reduction of mortality is 20% in most subgroups, this means that the number of lives saved is greatest in those at higher risk. So for example, the number of lives saved per 1000 patients treated is
49 in the presence of bundle branch block, 37 in the case of anterior myocardial infarction compared to only 8 in the case of inferior myocardial infarction. In the presence of diabetes 37 lives are saved compared to only 15 in the
absence of diabetes.

In the WARIS study warfarin given post-AMI reduced mortality by 24%,
recurrent AMI by 34% and CVAs by 55% at the cost of an annual severe
bleeding rate of 0.6%. Similar results were found in the ASPECT study but
there was only a 10% (NS) reduction in mortality. There have been no sub-
analyses in people with diabetes.

Aspirin, thienopyridines, and glycoprotein IIb/IIIa receptor inhibitors
Aspirin alone given as a dose of at least 150 mg soon after the onset of
symptoms of ACS and continued for at least a month reduced cardiovascular mortality by 20% compared to placebo. This represents benefit of 25
lives saved per 1000 treated patients. Reduction in re-infarction and non-
fatal CVAs are also reduced by almost 50%. Continuing the aspirin beyond

the first month doubles the initial benefit by preventing an additional 40 deaths, myocardial infarctions (MIs) or CVAs per 1000 treated patients during the first 4 years. The beneficial effects of aspirin and thrombolysis are additive and the streptokinase–aspirin combination has been shown to be the most effective regime with a 38% reduction of mortality. The benefits of aspirin in diabetics appear to be similar to those without diabetes although the optimum dose of aspirin remains to be determined.

In the general population, aspirin for primary prevention has been shown to reduce the number of non-fatal MIs and transient ischaemic attacks (TIAs) but with no effect on cardiovascular mortality. In some studies there was a suggestion of an increase in the number of haemorraghic strokes although this was not confirmed in the HOT study which suggested that, provided hypertension is well controlled, the addition of aspirin is beneficial. In practice, the treatment of 1000 high-risk subjects by aspirin for 1 year would prevent about three coronary ischaemic events. In people with diabetes, aspirin is indicated if the 10 years coronary heart disease (CHD) risk exceeds 15%.

Thienopyridines (ticlopidine and its derivative clopidogrel) do not inhibit cyclo-oxygenase like aspirin, but inhibit ADP-dependent binding of fibrinogen to IIb/IIIa glycoprotein receptors. Unfortunately, ticlopidine can cause neutropenia and thrombocytopaenia so has not been fully evaluated. Clopidogrel, on the other hand, both alone and in combination with aspirin has been shown to be superior to aspirin alone at reducing cardiovascular and cerebrovascular events. The benefits are small (an 8% difference compared to aspirin) however, and at today's prices it is not cost-effective. In the CURE study (Clopidogrel in Unstable Angina to Prevent Recurrent Ischaemic Events) over 12 000 patients (22% with diabetes) who presented within 24 hours of onset of symptoms of ACS, were randomized to receive aspirin 75–325 mg/day and either clopidogrel or placebo. There was a 20% reduction in events (9.28% vs. 11.47%) in the clopidogrel group and an 8% reduction in mortality. Thus, if clopidogrel has a place, it is in secondary prevention in those most at risk; this may include people with diabetes.

IIb/IIIa glycoprotein receptor inhibitors are powerful antiplatelet agents which if given to high risk patients with unstable angina or ACS, in conjunction with aspirin, reduce mortality and risk of MI. Studies in patients with diabetes suggest similar benefit. These agents are also useful following coronary angioplasty at reducing the risk of death and infarction.

Beta-blockers

Beta-blockers inhibit synthetic nervous system activity, reducing heart rate and decreasing myocardial oxygen consumption, so reducing ischaemia.

They also have antiarrhythmic effect and early i.v. administration has been shown to limit the size of myocardial damage. Many of the studies that were performed on beta blockade at the time of the infarct, and post infarction, were done in the prethrombolysis era. In combination with thrombolysis, intravenous beta-blockers, given early after the onset of symptoms, have been shown to significantly decrease recurrent angina and non-fatal recurrent MI during the first 6 days. Controversy remains over the mode of administration since the GUSTO-1 study showed that although overall mortality on the 30th day was significantly lower in patients treated with beta-blockers, i.v. administration worsened the prognosis compared to oral beta-blockers introduced after haemodynamic stabilization. Intravenous beta-blockers were associated with an increase in incidence of heart failure, shock and the need for ventricular pacing. A meta-analysis of data from 29 trials involving 29 000 patients on beta-blockers during MI showed a reduction in mortality of 13%. Pooled data from six trials conducted in patients with diabetes showed a 35% reduction in mortality. The benefits of beta-blockers given post MI (usually after a few days) have been analysed in another meta-analysis of some 24 000 patients and a 23% reduction in mortality was demonstrated. Diabetics had a greater benefit, however, of up to 48%.

Not all beta-blockers are the same, however, and only timolol, propranolol and metoprolol have been proven to be of value in these situations. Despite this, atenolol is the most popular beta-blocker in the UK.

For primary prevention of CHD events, beta-blockers appear to have no advantages over angiotensin-converting enzyme inhibitors (ACE-inhibitors) according to the UKPDS which compared Atenolol with captopril in the treatment of hypertension, though patients on Atenolol gained more weight (3.4 vs. 1.6 kg).

ACE inhibitors (ACE-I)

Studies have been conducted using ACE-Is acutely, at the time of MI or post MI. A meta-analysis of 15 acute trials with more than 100 000 patients showed a reduction in mortality of some 6%. This included the Consensus-2 trial using i.v. enalapril, in which there was an increased mortality of 11% in those treated with an ACE-I and a negative interaction with aspirin use was observed. In GISSI-3 patients who were hypotensive or in severe congestive cardiac failure were excluded and acute use of lisinopril was associated with a 6-week reduction in mortality of 44% in patients with type 1 diabetes and 27% in those with type 2 diabetes.

ACE-Is given post MI in patients with reduced left ventricular (LV) function show a reduction in mortality by 22% in patients with an LV ejection fraction of <40%. Similar reductions in mortality have been observed in patients with diabetes. The benefits of ACE-I observed in patients with LV dysfunction have subsequently been confirmed in high risk patients with normal LV function. In the Heart Outcomes Prevention Evaluation (HOPE) study, 9297 patients over the age of 55 years (mean age 66) with established vascular disease were randomized to receive ramipril 10 mg or placebo. Thirty-eight per cent ($n = 3578$) were diabetic (Micro-HOPE) and were followed for a mean of 4.5 years; treatment with ramipril was associated with a 24% reduction in all-cause mortality, 22% reduction in rate of MI and 33% reduction in rate of stroke (**Fig. 8.1**).

Treatment of hyperglycaemia

The DIGAMI study involved patients with an AMI and an admission blood glucose >11 mmol/l irrespective of their diabetes status. Patients were given a glucose/insulin infusion to maintain blood glucose control between 7 and 9 mmol/l followed by 3 months of four times daily subcutaneous insulin or assigned to the control group who received their usual treatment of diabetes (which might have included insulin if it were clinically indicated). A significant reduction in mortality of 29% was seen in the insulin/glucose infusion group compared to controls. The greatest benefit was seen in those at relatively low risk, i.e. younger patients not previously treated by insulin. They experienced a relative risk reduction of 52% at 1 year. Some authors have suggested that this increased benefit was related to discontinuation of oral antidiabetic agents such as sulphonylureas but this seems unlikely as the UKPDS study showed no difference in mortality between those treated with sulphonylureas and insulin.

Revascularization

Urgent revascularization is usually undertaken in refractory unstable angina that fails to settle despite optimum medical therapy. In 90–95% of patients, medical therapy stabilizes the situation. Early intervention, with angiography and angioplasty where appropriate, has not been shown to be superior to medical treatment alone.

IIb/IIIa glycoprotein receptor inhibitors improve the prognosis of patients treated by coronary angioplasty, but medical therapy alone has a similar or better prognosis. Surgery and angioplasty have similar results— vein grafting only improves prognosis in patients with triple vessel disease or LV dysfunction. There is no evidence that diabetics need an alternative strategy except that the BARI study suggested that people with diabetes did less well with angioplasty—this remains to be confirmed. The role of other antiplatelet agents such as clopidogrel, or angioplasty followed by stenting remains uncertain.

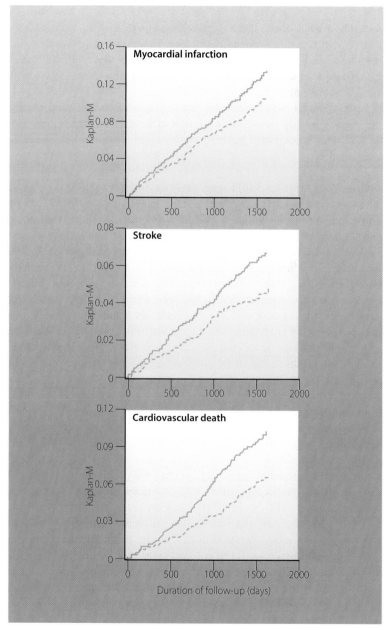

Fig. 8.1 Effects of ramipril on cardiovascular outcomes in people with diabetes—Micro-HOPE. *Lancet 2000;* **355**: 253–9.

Statins

Statins have transformed the management of hyperlipidaemia reducing both total mortality, coronary events and need for revascularization. What is clear is that this is not due to cholesterol lowering alone. They have significant anti-inflammatory effects reducing C-reactive protein (CRP) and probably stabilize atheromatous plaques.

Several clinical trials have now looked at the effect of initiating a statin within hours and days of a coronary event and the findings suggest there may be significant benefits. The RECIFE (Reduction of Cholesterol in Ischaemia and Function of the Endothelium) trial looked at the effect of rapidly lowering cholesterol on endothelial function days after a coronary event. Patients admitted with MI or unstable angina were randomized to placebo or pravastatin 40 mg within 10 days. Endothelial function was assessed by measuring flow-mediated dilatation of the brachial artery, which increased by 42% with pravastatin compared with placebo. More excitingly, other short-term studies with pravastatin 40 mg and atorvastatin 80 mg initiated within 4 days have shown significant reductions in coronary events in as little as 16 weeks. Larger trials are on-going which will help to determine if these preliminary findings are confirmed and if this is a class effect. Not all statins have been demonstrated to lower CRP, and smooth muscle cell proliferation (which may help stablize plaques) is inhibited by some statins *in vivo* but not by pravastatin.

Potential but unproven interventions such as use of antioxidants, treatment of homocysteinaemia (with folic acid) or hypertriglyceridaemia remain untested. In the HOPE study vitamin E conferred no benefit.

Peripheral vascular disease

The Wisconsin Epidemiological Study of Diabetic Retinopathy (WESDR) included nearly 3000 people with diabetes (1200 type 1 patients diagnosed under 30 years) and showed an association between rising $HbA1_C$ and risk of lower limb amputation. However, neither the Diabetes Control and Complications Trial (DCCT) nor UKPDS were powered to look at peripheral vascular disease (PVD) or an amputation as an end-point—DCCT patients were young and few had macrovascular events; UKPDS patients with significant peripheral vascular disease at diagnosis were excluded from the study. There was a non-significant (16%) reduction in fatal and non-fatal MIs in the intensively treated group after 15 years and there was no difference between the intensive and conventional treatment groups in the proportion of patients who had evidence of PVD by Doppler blood pressure or absent peripheral pulses. No control-led trials have been undertaken with diabetic patients to assess the effects of risk factor modification on the regression of vascular disease, however, smoking cessation is associated with improvement of symptoms in non-diabetics. Among patients with symptomatic PVD, continued smoking is associated with worsening claudication, limb-threatening ischaemia and amputation, and the need for revascularization. Patency rates are lower following revascularization in patients who continue to smoke and survival is reduced. The effects of management of hyperlipidaemia and hypertension on the progression of PVD has not been fully evaluated but an analysis of the Scandanavian Simvastatin Survival Study (4S) showed that the incidence of 'new or worsening, claudication' was significantly lower in CHD patients treated with Simvastatin (**Fig. 8.2**). In the Physician's Health study, low doses of aspirin resulted in a 54% reduction in the risk of peripheral arterial surgery, compared with placebo, but no study has shown any improvement in claudication symptoms with antiplatelet agents. Drug treatment for claudication has generally been disappointing but a new agent, cilostazol (a phosphodiesterase III inhibitor with antiplatelet, antithrombotic and vasodilatory effects), looks promising. Phase III studies involving just over 2000 patients (approximately 25% with diabetes) using doses of between 50 and 100 mg twice daily, showed improvement in maximal walking distance in most but not all studies. Pain-free walking distance and quality of life were improved and Cilostazol was significantly better than both placebo and oxpentifylline 400 mg tid (**Fig. 8.3**).

Peripheral vascular disease is a contributory factor in most diabetic foot ulcers, and evidence exists that a combination of a dedicated multidisciplinary

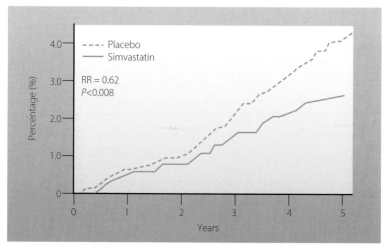

Fig. 8.2 Effect of simvastatin on incidence of 'new or worsening' intermittent claudication in the Scandinavian Simvastatin Survival (4S) study. *Am J Cardiol* 1998; **81**: 333–5.

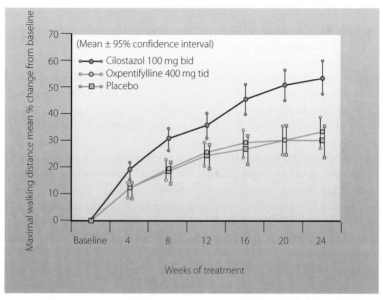

Fig. 8.3 Maximal walking distance in patients with claudication treated with Cilostazol or pentoxifylline or placebo. *Circulation* 1998; **98** (Suppl 1): 1012, Abstract 58.

foot service and the utilization of specialist footwear can reduce both ulceration and amputation rates.

Cerebrovascular disease

In UKPDS each 1% reduction in $HbA1_C$ was associated with a 37% decrease in risk for microvascular complications and a 21% decrease in the risk of any diabetes-related end-point or death. The association with glycaemia was less steep for stroke and heart failure (**Fig. 8.4**), for which hypertension is a much more important contributory factor but nevertheless improved glycaemia reduced the incidence of stroke. Unfortunately, acute stroke management in the person with diabetes is based on extrapolation of the data from non-diabetics as there are, as yet, no prospective studies of stroke management in diabetics. Trials have shown that thrombolytic therapy started within 6 hours of the onset of symptoms of ischaemic stroke reduces the proportion of patients who die or remain dependent on others, up to 6 months later (61.5% vs. 68% of control patients not given thrombolysis). Results were more impressive if treatment was started within 3 hours (56.6% vs. 70.7%). Alteplase seemed superior to streptokinase but overall there was an increased risk of symptomatic intracranial haemorrhage (9.6% vs. 2.6%). Overall, the risk of dying within 2 weeks was increased in those receiv-

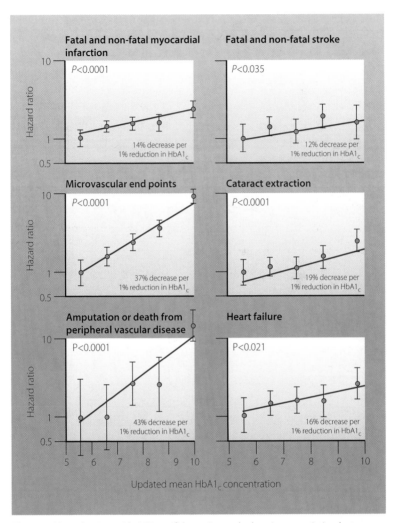

Fig. 8.4 Hazard ratios, with 95% confidence intervals showing association between mean HbA1$_c$ and various micro- and macrovascular complications in the UKPDS trial. *BMJ* 2000; **321**: 405–412, with permission.

ing thrombolytic therapy (20.9% vs. 11.9%) despite the improvement in the composite end-point of death or dependency. Whether people with diabetes benefit similarly from thrombolysis is not known. Use of anticoagulant therapy with unfractionated or low-molecular weight heparin for acute ischaemic stroke is associated with an increase in haemorrhagic stroke but with no positive benefit in terms of mortality or dependency.

Hyperglycaemia on admission is associated with a worse outcome and although the benefits of treatment of hyperglycaemia in this situation are unknown, a DIGAMI-style glucose and insulin infusion would seem sensible (trials are ongoing).

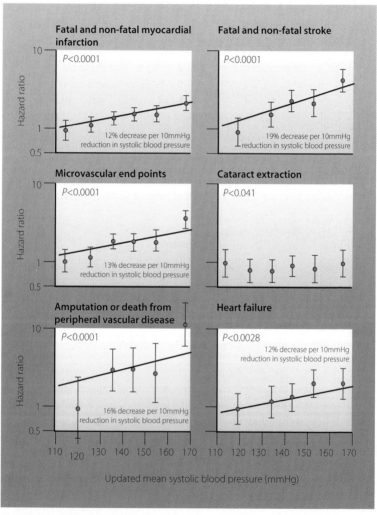

Fig. 8.5 Hazard ratios (95%) confidence intervals) showing association between mean systolic blood pressure and various micro- and macrovascular complications in the UKPDS study. *BMJ* 2000; **321**: 413–17, with permission.

Secondary prevention data is based entirely on general population studies with none having been conducted in people with diabetes alone. Targets similar for those of diabetic patients with CHD are appropriate. The dose of aspirin required is uncertain. The European Stroke Prevention Study showed that, in the general population, aspirin and sustained-release dipyridamole are equally effective secondary prevention in reducing the risk of stroke and/or death. However, doubts exist because of the relatively low dose of aspirin used and the exclusion of one centre from the study because of scientific fraud. In the Clopidogrel vs. Aspirin in Patients at Risk of Ischaemic Events (CAPRIE) study 7.2% of those treated with clopidogrel 75 mg/day had an event compared with 7.7% of patients receiving aspirin 325 mg/day. So, if the patient has a cerebrovascular incident whilst on aspirin addition of dipyridamole may be justified; where patients have a true aspirin allergy clopidogrel is probably the most appropriate choice.

There are number of studies where stroke prevention has been a significant secondary end-point. The UKPDS hypertension study, where the target for tight blood pressure control was <150/85, showed a 44% reduction in strokes compared to the less tight blood pressure control group (target blood pressure < 180/105) (**Fig. 8.5**).

Ramipril 10 mg daily in the diabetic subgroup (Micro-HOPE) of the HOPE study reduced the number of strokes from 6.1% to 4.2% (a 33% relative risk reduction) in a cohort of patients most of whom had established CHD. The difference in blood pressure between the ramipril and placebo groups at the end of the study was only 2.5/1.0—some commentators say this is insufficient to account for the difference in stroke rates, but as these were based on casual readings rather than 24-hour profiles it remains uncertain whether the benefit is due to blood pressure lowering or a different mode of vascular protection by ACE-Is.

In both CARE and LIPID (secondary prevention studies in patients with previous MI or angina), pravastatin 40 mg reduced the risk of fatal and non-fatal cerebrovascular accidents by 31% and 20%, respectively—the numbers with diabetes, however, were too small to analyse as a separate group.

Nephropathy

The DCCT showed a 39% reduction in the occurrence of microalbuminuria and a 54% reduction in albuminuria in the intensive therapy arm for both adults and adolescents with type 1 diabetes. Similarly, the UKPDS showed a slowing of renal decline in the tight glycaemic control group with type 2 diabetes (**Fig. 8.6**). Type 2 patients with microalbuminuria or proteinuria are less likely to progress to end-stage renal failure (ESRF) but as with type 1 diabetes, blood pressure management is the mainstay of treatment to reduce the decline in renal function. ACE-Is are indicated in type 1 patients with persistent microalbuminuria or proteinuria, irrespective of initial blood pressure (**Fig. 8.7**) and are first-line agents in type 2 diabetes if microalbuminuria or

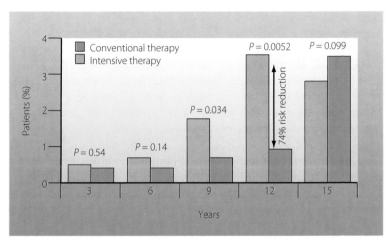

Fig. 8.6 Effect of glycaemic control on creatinine increase in UK Prospective Diabetes Study Group. From *Lancet* 1998; **352**: 837–53.

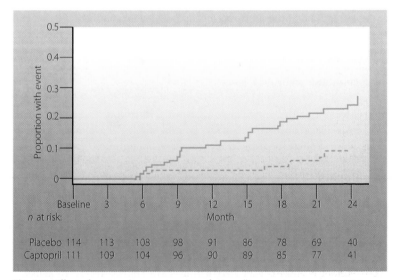

Fig. 8.7 Effect of captopril on progression of microalbuminuria in normotensive patients with type 1 diabetes. *Diabetologia* 1996; **39**: 587–93.

proteinuria is present though lowering blood pressure is the priority. Renoprotection by ACE-Is is probably a class effect. To achieve a target blood pressure of <130/80 for patients with nephropathy may require several antihypertensive agents and for young people BP targets may be set even lower to achieve a BP <90th centile for age.

Retinopathy

The DCCT demonstrated beyond doubt that good glycaemic control retarded the onset of microvascular complications and delayed progression of those complications already present. Almost a half of patients in the intensive treatment arm achieved an $HbA1_C$ of 6.1% or less at least once during the study to give a mean of approximately 7% for the duration of the study. From 5 years into the study there was a 50% reduction in the cumulative incidence of retinopathy in the primary prevention cohort and a 54% reduction in progression in the secondary prevention arm compared to the conventional treatment group (mean $HbA1_C$ 8.9%) (**Figs 8.8 and 8.9**). Intensive therapy

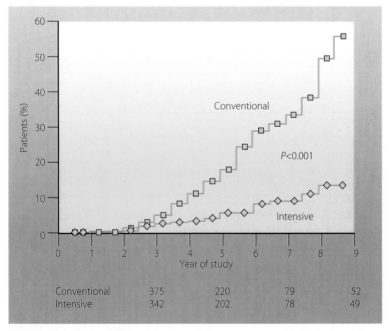

Fig. 8.8 Cumulative incidence of sustained change in retinopathy in patients with IDDM receiving intensive or conventional therapy in the primary prevention arm of the DCCT. Year of study refers to sample sizes at different years of the study. *NEJM* 1993; **329**: 977–86.

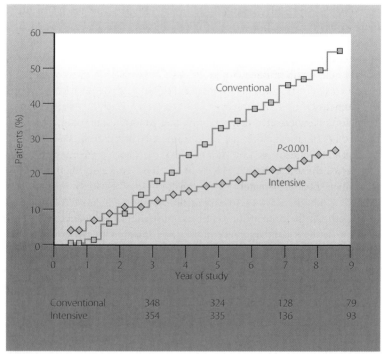

Fig. 8.9 Cumulative incidence of sustained change in retinopathy in patients with IDDM receiving intensive or conventional therapy in the secondary prevention arm of the DCCT. Year of study refers to sample sizes at different years of the study. *NEJM* 1993; **329**: 977–86.

reduced the risk of preproliferative and proliferative retinopathy by 47% and need for photocoagulation by 56%.

In the UKPDS, hypertensive patients were assigned to either tight or moderate blood pressure control over 9 years. The group randomized to tight blood pressure control (mean 144/82 mmHg) experienced a 47% reduction in the risk of losing three lines of vision compared to the group with standard blood pressure control (mean 154/87 mmHg). There was also a 34% reduction in the risk of progression of retinopathy status. The EURODIAB Controlled Trial of Lisinopril in Insulin-Dependent Diabetes Mellitus (EUCLID), also comparing tight with moderate blood pressure control, produced similar results, i.e. a significantly reduced risk of blindness and reduced rate of progression of retinopathy in those patients randomized to more intensively controlled blood pressure. Use of an ACE-I may reduce the progression of retinopathy, independently of blood pressure reduction, especially in normotensive type 1 diabetics.

Neuropathy

In the primary prevention cohort of the DCCT, intensive therapy delayed the appearance of neuropathy at 5 years by 69%. Ten per cent of the conventional treatment group developed neuropathy compared to 3% in the conventional group. Progression (as judged by clinical findings and nerve conduction studies) was reduced by 59%.

In UKPDS, however, no differences were observed between treatment groups. Aldose reductase inhibitors have not been found to give sustained or clinically relevant improvements in nerve function

CONCLUSION

The last two decades have seen the publication of a large number of well designed, randomized controlled trials which have identified interventions that can prevent or retard the progression of the micro- and macrovascular complications of diabetes. The combination of intensified glycaemic control, and aggressive treatment of hypertension and hyperlipidaemia offers the person with diabetes the chance to extend life-expectancy and improve quality of life. Health organizations, pharmaceutical companies and politicians must work closely together to devise strategies aimed at preventing type 2 diabetes and setting up health surveillance systems that identify patients early in their disease—prior to the onset of complications, so that these interventions can have the maximum benefit. Nevertheless, these treatments require great commitment from both patient and health professionals and are for most of the world's diabetic population, at present, unaffordable.

FURTHER READING

Klein R. Hyperglycaemia and microvascular and macrovascular disease in diabetes. *Diabetes Care* 1995; **18**(2) 258–68.

The Diabetes Control and Complications Trial Research Group. The effect of intensive treatment of diabetes on the development and progression of long-term complications in insulin dependent diabetes mellitus. *NEJM* 1993; **329**: 977–86.

UK Prospective Diabetes Study (UKPDS) Group. Intensive blood-glucose control with sulphonylureas or insulin compared with conventional treatment and risk of complications in patients with type 2 diabetes (UKPDS 33). *Lancet* 1998; **352**: 837–53.

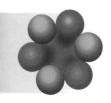

DIABETIC RETINOPATHY AND ASSOCIATED OPHTHALMIC DISORDERS

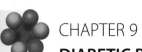

CHAPTER 9
DIABETIC RETINOPATHY: EPIDEMIOLOGY AND RISK FACTORS

INTRODUCTION

The annual rate of blind registration due to diabetic retinopathy appears to be falling in some European countries, but diabetes remains the leading cause of blindness in the working age group, accounting for approximately 12% of all cases of registrable blindness among those <65 years old. The incidence of visual impairment during a 4-year observation period has been best documented by the Wisconsin Epidemiologic Study of Diabetic Retinopathy (WESDR), a large population-based study conducted in 10 counties in southern Wisconsin, USA (**Table 9.1**). Approximately 10% of all diabetic patients in primary care were examined and followed-up. The subjects were divided into two groups: those with an age of onset of diabetes below 30 years and those with an age of onset above 30 years. This latter group was further subdivided into those treated with insulin and those not taking insulin. Subjects were re-examined at several time points (4 and 10 years) to document the incidence and prevalence of diabetic retinopathy and the associated risk factors.

In the WESDR, visual impairment was subdivided into four categories ranging from none to blind and data at baseline was compared with that 4 years later (**Table 9.1**). For example, in the 832 younger onset (i.e. <30 years) subjects with no visual impairment at baseline, 2.8%, 1.4% and 0.5% had progressed to mild impairment, moderate impairment and blindness respectively by 4 years (**Table 9.1**).

BLINDNESS RATES IN DIABETIC PATIENTS

The annual incidence of blindness from diabetic retinopathy varies between 0.02 and 1%, and the prevalence of blindness in diabetic patients is approximately 2%. Diabetic retinopathy accounts for between 8 and 12% of all registrable blindness (defined as a Snellen visual acuity of 6/60 or worse in the better eye).

PREVALENCE OF DIABETIC RETINOPATHY

Summary of findings from the WESDR:

Onset of diabetes before age 30 years (**Fig. 9.1**):
- The prevalence of any retinopathy is 2% in those within 2 years of diagnosis of diabetes and 98% in those with disease duration >15 years.
- The prevalence of proliferative retinopathy is 0% in those within 5 years of diagnosis of diabetes, rising to 67% in those with disease duration >35 years.

Onset of diabetes after age 30 years (**Fig. 9.2**):
- The prevalence of any retinopathy is 29% in those within 5 years of diagnosis of diabetes and 78% in those with disease duration >15 years.
- The prevalence of proliferative retinopathy is 2% in those within 5 years of onset of diabetes, rising to 16% in those with disease duration >15 years.

The higher prevalence of retinopathy in those diagnosed with diabetes over the age of 30 is partly due to the difficulty in determining the precise date of onset of disease. The prevalence of retinopathy at the time of diagnosis of type 2 diabetes has been reported to be as high as 38%.

Four-year Incidence of Visual Impairment in Participants Surviving and Completing the Follow-up Examination					
Visual impairment at baseline	Number of participants	None (%)	Mild (%)	Moderate (%)	Blind (%)
*Younger onset**					
None	832	95.3	2.8	1.4	0.5
Mild	26	26.9	42.3	15.4	15.4
Moderate	10	10.0	10.0	30.0	50.0
Blind	20	0	0	0	100.0
Older-onset, taking insulin †					
None	423	83.9	10.6	4.3	1.2
Mild	27	29.6	22.6	40.7	7.4
Moderate	15	6.7	13.3	26.7	53.3
Blind	8	0	0	0	100.0
Older onset, not taking insulin §					
None	454	91.0	5.5	2.9	0.7
Mild	29	20.7	31.0	31.0	17.2
Moderate	7	0	0	28.6	71.4
Blind	4	0	0	0	100.0

* In three persons the baseline and/or follow-up impairment level could not be determined.
† In 12 persons, the baseline and/or follow-up impairment level could not be determined.

Table 9.1 Four-year incidence of visual impairment in participants surviving and completing the follow-up examination. Derived from the Wisconsin Epidemiologic Study of Diabetic Retinopathy (WESDR). The levels of visual acuity were classified as: no impairment (better than 20/40), mild impairment (20/40–20/63), moderate impairment (20/80–20/160) and blind (≥20/200). *Ophthalmology* 1988; **95**: 1340–8.

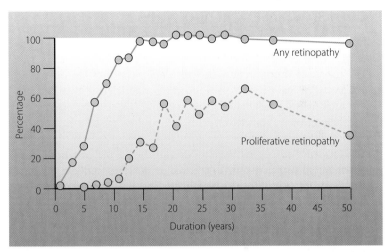

Fig. 9.1 Frequency of any retinopathy and prolifereative retinopathy by duration of diabetes in type I diabetes. Derived from the Wisconsin Epidemiologic Study of Diabetic Retinopathy (WESDR). *Arch Ophthalmol* 1984; **102**: 520–6.

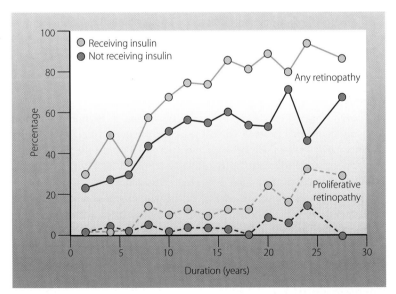

Fig. 9.2 Frequency of any retinopathy and prolifereative retinopathy by duration of diabetes in patients with type 2 diabetes, according to insulin status. Derived from the Wisconsin Epidemiologic Study of Diabetic Retinopathy (WESDR). *Arch Ophthalmol* 1984; **102**: 527–32.

INCIDENCE OF DIABETIC RETINOPATHY

Summary of findings from the WESDR:

Onset of diabetes before age 30:

- The incidence of any retinopathy developing for the first time over a 4-year and 10-year period is 59% and 90%, respectively.
- The incidence of proliferative retinopathy over a 4-year and 10-year period is 11% and 30%, respectively.

Onset of diabetes after age 30:

- The incidence of any retinopathy developing for the first time over a 4-year and 10-year period is 34–47% and 67–80%, respectively.
- The incidence of proliferative retinopathy over a 4-year and 10-year period is 2–7% and 10–23%, respectively.

RISK FACTORS FOR DIABETIC RETINOPATHY

Hyperglycaemia

Chronic hyperglycaemia is the major risk factor in the development of diabetic retinopathy. The US Diabetes Control and Complications Trial (DCCT) evaluated the rates of development of microvascular complications in two groups of type 1 diabetics assigned either to strict or standard glycaemic control over a mean follow-up period of 6.5 years. Those who had no retinopathy at entry into the study and who were assigned to tight control showed a 76% reduction in the mean risk of developing retinopathy. In addition, among those subjects with mild retinopathy at baseline, tight control slowed the progression of retinopathy by 54% and reduced the likelihood of severe or proliferative retinopathy by 47%.

The UK Prospective Diabetes Study (UKPDS) similarly examined the effect of tight vs. standard glycaemic control in newly diagnosed patients with type 2 diabetes. Over 10 years, $HbA1_C$ levels averaged 11% lower in the tight control group, which resulted in a 25% risk reduction in microvascular complications, including the need for panretinal laser photocoagulation.

The WESDR examined the 4-year incidence and progression of retinopathy in relation to $HbA1_C$ and showed that patients in the highest quartile of $HbA1_C$ experienced the greatest incidence and progression of retinopathy (**Fig. 9.3**). It is estimated that by reducing $HbA1_C$ from 11% to 9% the rate of progression to proliferative disease would be halved.

Duration of diabetes

Duration of diabetes is a reliable predictor of the presence of retinopathy, but the severity of the retinopathy is primarily influenced by other risk factors, especially glycaemic control.

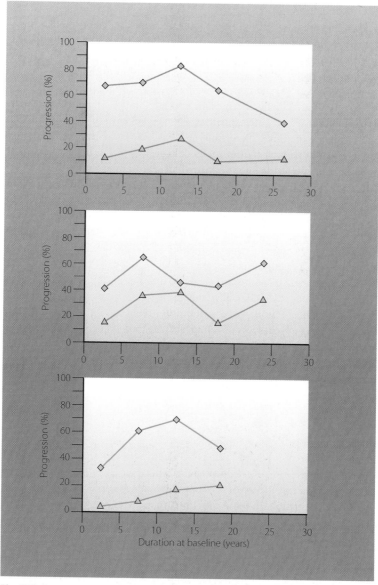

Fig. 9.3 Four-year progression of retinopathy by quartile of HbA1$_c$ and duration of diabetes at baseline in persons with (top) younger-onset diabetes; (centre) older-onset diabetes, taking insulin; and (bottom) older-onset diabetes, not taking insulin. △ indicate first quartile; ◇, fourth quartile. Derived from Wisconsin Epidemiologic Study of Diabetic Retinopathy. *JAMA* 1988; **260**: 2864–71.

Blood pressure

High blood pressure (BP) is a major independent risk factor in the development of retinopathy in both type 1 and type 2 diabetes. Even among relatively normotensive individuals (BP <140/90 mmHg), those with BP levels above the 90th percentile show a higher prevalence of retinopathy and higher rate of progression. Hypertension is roughly twice as common in diabetic compared with non-diabetic patients. For example, 17–24% of patients with type 1 diabetes and 38% of patients with type 2 diabetes have BP >160/90 mmHg.

Because of the link between BP and diabetic renal complications, it has been difficult to establish from epidemiological work that hypertension is an independent risk factor for retinopathy but several intervention studies have been conclusive. In the UKPDS, hypertensive patients were assigned to either tight or moderate BP control over 9 years. The group randomized to tight BP control (mean 144/82 mmHg) experienced a 47% reduction in the risk of losing three lines of vision compared to the group with standard BP control (mean BP 154/87 mmHg). There was also a 34% reduction in the risk of progression of retinopathy status.

The EURODIAB Controlled Trial of Lisinopril in Insulin-Dependent Diabetes Mellitus (EUCLID), also comparing tight with moderate BP control, produced similar results, i.e. a significantly reduced risk of blindness and reduced rate of progression of retinopathy in those patients randomized to more intensively controlled BP. Use of an angiotensin converting enzyme-inhibitor (ACE-I) may be particularly effective in reducing the progression of retinopathy, independently of BP reduction, especially in normotensive type 1 diabetics.

Age

Diabetic retinopathy is rare under 10 years of age; only one case was seen in the first decade of life in the WESDR. Puberty, with its attendant hormonal changes, brings about accelerated changes in retinopathy status; the highest 4-year incidence in the WESDR was among patients aged 10–12 years at the baseline examination. In those with onset of diabetes below 21 years, females developed retinopathy approximately 2 years ahead of males, once again suggesting a pubertal influence.

Nephropathy

Patients with diabetic nephropathy are much more likely to have associated microvascular disease in the eye; up to 96% of those with nephropathy also have retinopathy. In type 2 diabetes, microalbuminuria is an independent predictor of retinopathy. This suggests similar pathogenic mechanisms, but a significant proportion of patients with advanced retinopathy show no clinical evidence of nephropathy. Similarly, although unusual, advanced renal disease has been described in the absence of retinopathy. It therefore seems likely that each form of microvascular disease has overlapping but not identical pathogenic mechanisms. Beyond its predictive value, nephropathy may also signify the presence of a more severe form of retinopathy, one that is more resistant to the effects of laser therapy.

Plasma lipids

The role of plasma lipids in the development of diabetic retinopathy is unclear. In the WESDR, baseline serum cholesterol level had no relationship with retinopathy status 5 years later in type 1 diabetics. Other studies, however, have suggested an association between higher levels of total serum cholesterol, declining ratios of high density lipoprotein (HDL) cholesterol/total cholesterol and more severe retinopathy. As part of the Sorbinil Retinopathy Trial in type 1 diabetes, total serum cholesterol was found to have a marginal effect on the rate of progression of retinopathy. In a small case-control study of type 2 diabetic patients by Dodson and Gibson, patients with maculopathy were followed-up over 7 years and compared with a matched group of patients without maculopathy. The group with maculopathy was found to have higher serum cholesterol levels (6.6 vs. 5.9 mmol/l), higher levels of the HDL2 subfraction (0.46 vs. 0.32 mmol/l) and a higher prevalence of hyperlipidaemia (54% vs. 35%).

The Early Treatment Diabetic Retinopathy Study (ETDRS) group reported that patients with persistently poor vision had higher blood cholesterol levels. They also found that patients with high total cholesterol and LDL-cholesterol had twice the number of retinal hard exudates compared with those with normal lipid levels; the risk of losing vision was related to the extent of hard exudates, even after adjusting for macular oedema. These patients also developed more hard exudates during the course of the study. This finding is supported by the WESDR, which also reported an association between higher cholesterol levels and the extent of retinal hard exudation.

Genetic factors

It seems likely that there is a component of inherited susceptibility to the various microvascular complications of diabetes, because some individuals appear not to develop retinopathy despite poor glycaemic control. Familial clustering of diabetic retinopathy was investigated among 372 subjects with type 1 diabetes in the DCCT. The presence and severity of retinopathy was assessed in first-degree diabetic relatives of subjects in the trial. The severity of retinopathy in parents of children probands was found to be linked with the severity of retinopathy in their children, with the link strongest between mother and child. However, no relationship could be established between siblings. Although this observation suggests that the severity of diabetic retinopathy may be influenced by familial factors, the difficulty remains in differentiating environmental from genetic influences.

Pregnancy

Diabetic retinopathy often gets worse during pregnancy, but it has been difficult to demonstrate that the progression of retinopathy is related to the pregnancy and would not otherwise have occurred. The issue has recently been clarified by two case-control studies. Moloney and Drury studied the progression of retinopathy prospectively in two groups of diabetic women who were matched apart from pregnancy status. The pregnant group demonstrated both increased prevalence and severity of retinopathy status compared to the control group. This finding is further supported by a larger study where the rate of progression of retinopathy was also found to be greater in the pregnant group after accounting for the influence of duration of diabetes, glycaemic control and hypertension.

The Diabetes in Early Pregnancy Study reported that the risk of progression of retinopathy is greatest in women with moderate to severe retinopathy at the start of the pregnancy; for example, 29% of subjects with moderate retinopathy at baseline developed proliferative features, compared with 6% of those with minimal retinopathy at baseline. The study also found that women with the highest glycosylated haemoglobin levels at the start of pregnancy, and those who experienced the greatest improvement in glycaemic control during pregnancy, had the highest risk of progression of retinopathy status. This may be one major reason why retinopathy progresses during pregnancy, since retinopathy status can temporarily deteriorate after institution of tight glycaemic control; aiming for improved glycaemic control during pregnancy features strongly in the antenatal care of diabetic patients.

Although current pregnancy may adversely affect retinopathy status, it has been reported that in the long term parous women have a lower prevalence of any retinopathy and of severe retinopathy. This may be the consequence of the institution of better control during pregnancy continuing into the postpartum period.

Ophthalmic supervision is therefore important during pregnancy particularly when retinopathy status at the start of pregnancy is moderately advanced. Those women with poor glycaemic control at the start of pregnancy also require close supervision.

Ocular factors

It has been observed that patients with asymmetrical diabetic retinopathy have a higher ophthalmic arterial perfusion pressure in the more severely affected eye. Ocular perfusion pressure is associated with the incidence of retinopathy. Higher intraocular pressure (therefore lower perfusion pressure) may offer some protection against retinopathy. Other factors found to be associated with a reduced risk of retinopathy include myopia, extensive chorioretinal scarring (perhaps simulating the effects of panretinal laser treatment) and amblyopia.

CURRENT ISSUES

- The incidence of blindness from diabetic retinopathy appears to have been diminishing over the last two decades, but diabetic eye disease remains the leading cause of registrable blindness in the working age group (accounting for 12% of all cases).
- The principal risk factor in the development of diabetic retinopathy is that of hyperglycaemia; it has now been definitively shown that tight glycaemic control reduces the incidence and progression of retinopathy. Sudden improvements in glycaemic control may, however, worsen retinopathy during the first year but any adverse effect is usually transient.
- Intensive BP control reduces the risk of progression of retinopathy. Even small reductions in BP translate into large clinical benefits.

FURTHER READING

Diabetes Control and Complications Trial Research Group. The effect of intensive treatment of diabetes on the development and progression of long-term complications in insulin-dependent diabetes. *N Engl J Med* 1993; **329**: 977–986.

Klein, R, Klein BEK, Moss SE, Davis MD, DeMets KL. The Wisconsin Epidemiologic Study of Diabetic Retinopathy. II. Prevalence and risk of diabetic retinopathy when age at diagnosis is less than 30 years. *Arch Ophthalmol* 1984; **102**: 520–526.

Klein, R, Klein BEK, Moss SE, Davis MD, DeMets KL. The Wisconsin Epidemiologic Study of Diabetic Retinopathy. III. Prevalence and risk of diabetic retinopathy when age at diagnosis is 30 or more years. *Arch Ophthalmol* 1984; **102**: 527–532.

UK Prospective Diabetes Study (UKPDS) Group. Intensive blood-glucose control with sulphonylureas or insulin compared with conventional treatment and risk of complications in patients with type 2 diabetes (UKPDS 33). *Lancet* 1998; **352**: 837–853.

UK Prospective Diabetes Study (UKPDS) Group. Tight blood pressure control and risk of macrovascular and microvascular complications in type 2 diabetes: UKPDS 38. BMJ 1998; **317**: 703–13.

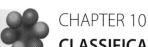

CHAPTER 10

CLASSIFICATION AND DIAGNOSIS OF DIABETIC RETINOPATHY

Hean-Choon Chen FRCS, FRCOpath

INTRODUCTION

The clinical features of diabetic retinopathy result from pathological changes within the retinal vasculature which are classified into two principal stages: background retinopathy and proliferative retinopathy. Background retinopathy has also been referred to as non-proliferative retinopathy to differentiate it from proliferative retinopathy although the proliferative changes occur amongst the 'background' of non-proliferative features. The terms most commonly used to denote the various stages of diabetic retinopathy are: background retinopathy, preproliferative retinopathy (a subclassification within background retinopathy) and proliferative retinopathy.

BACKGROUND DIABETIC RETINOPATHY

Background diabetic retinopathy is common and ranges from the very earliest signs of retinopathy to the severe changes seen just before the development of proliferative retinopathy. For practical purposes, background retinopathy can be subclassified into two subgroups of patients: those with sight-threatening disease and those without. The patterns of retinopathy most likely to reduce vision are those with macular involvement (maculopathy) and preproliferative disease (Table 10.1). Maculopathy denotes the lesions of background disease within the macular area, whereas prepoliferative retinopathy has additional features which differentiate it from the lesions of less severe background retinopathy. The three basic lesions which make up background retinopathy are microaneurysms, retinal haemorrhages and exudates. Haemorrhages and exudates have a limited lifespan, and, to a lesser extent, this also applies to microaneurysms.

Stages of diabetic retinopathy		
Background	Non-sight threatening	Microaneurysms, haemorrhages, exudates
Maculopathy	Cotton wool spots, large intraretinal haemorrhages, intraretinal vascular abnormalities (IRMA)	
Pre-proliferative	Venous abnormalities (beading, duplication, loops)	
Proliferative	New vessels, fibrovascular tissue, retinal detachment, vitreous haemorrhage	

Table 10.1 Stages of diabetic retinopathy.

Microaneurysms

These are the very earliest clinically detectable lesions of diabetic retinopathy (**Fig. 10.1**). They appear as small, round, red dots and may be found in any part of the retina although they predominate in the posterior pole of the eye. They are not associated with any visible blood vessels and represent localized dilatations of retinal capillaries. The number of microaneurysms increases with increasing severity of retinopathy. A microaneurysm indicates a localized area in the microvascular circulation where the blood–retinal barrier is deficient and may therefore be associated with abnormal vascular leakage.

The pathogenesis of microaneurysms is unclear but they may represent outpouchings of capillaries at areas of relative weakness where there is pericyte loss. Pericytes are cells which partly enclose retinal capillaries and may be considered the smooth muscle equivalent of the microvasculature; pericyte numbers diminish early in the development of diabetic retinopathy. Microaneurysms may also represent a localized response to surrounding hypoxia, i.e. a limited proliferative process, as they tend to predominate in areas where there is closure of surrounding capillary beds.

Haemorrhages

Haemorrhages coexist with microaneurysms but are more variable in their appearance (**Fig. 10.1**). At their smallest, they may be difficult to differentiate from microaneurysms. A haemorrhage, unlike a microaneurysm, is not

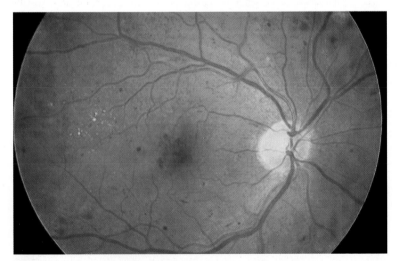

Fig. 10.1 Moderate background diabetic retinopathy with microaneurysms, haemorrhages and exudates.

necessarily round and may take on a variety of outlines; the phrase 'dot and blot' is an apt description. Haemorrhages can occur within the retina, where they remain confined by the retina, or they can occur on the retinal surface (flame-shaped haemorrhage) where they spread out over the superficial nerve fibre layer taking on a characteristic flame appearance. This latter form of haemorrhage is less obviously a feature of diabetic retinopathy and may suggest the coexistence of hypertensive vessel damage.

Haemorrhages probably occur from rupture of microaneurysms or other weak-walled vascular abnormalities. Small intraretinal haemorrhages occur early in diabetic retinopathy and their numbers increase with increasing severity. In more advanced disease, large dark blot intraretinal haemorrhages suggest severe retinal ischaemia with arteriolar occlusion, a feature of pre-proliferative disease.

Exudates

These are usually small collections of lipoprotein which have accumulated within the retina from abnormal vascular leakage, and are therefore found in the vicinity of microaneurysms (**Fig. 10.1**). They are usually reflective and may appear to have a rigid, multifaceted contour, ranging in colour from white to yellow. They were previously referred to as 'hard' exudates to differentiate them from soft exudates (now called cotton wool spots); however, this separation is now redundant since it is well established that cotton wool spots are not the products of exudation.

Like microaneurysms, exudates are most frequently detected in the posterior pole and may be distributed in the form of a whole or partial ring appearance (**Fig. 10.2**). Such 'circinate' ring arrangements usually have microaneurysms in the centre, which are responsible for the vascular leakage that gives rise to the exudates at the margins. The number of exudates may paradoxically increase as the degree of extravascular fluid diminishes due to precipitation of lipids and proteins, analogous to a saline solution depositing salt upon drying. There may therefore be a transient increase in the number of exudates following laser treatment as the macula becomes drier.

What is diabetic maculopathy?

The term macula refers to the important centre of the retina. It measures approximately 5 mm in diameter and is the area centred upon the fovea with a radius that extends to the temporal margin of the optic disc. The fovea itself is about the same size as the optic disc (1.5–1.7 mm in diameter), with its centre (foveola) recognizable in normal eyes by the foveolar reflex. More practically, the macula can be considered as the area within the major temporal vascular arcades.

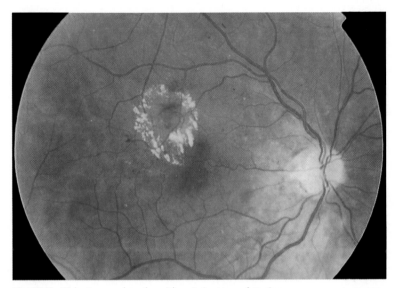

Fig. 10.2   Diabetic maculopathy with a circinate exudate ring.

Diabetic maculopathy can be defined as any retinopathy lesion located within the macula. However, the term maculopathy is usually reserved for sight-threatening lesions close to the centre of the macula. The Early Treatment Diabetic Retinopathy Study (ETDRS) group produced the following list of criteria, any one of which is sufficient to diagnose clinically significant macular oedema (CSMO) requiring laser treatment:

· Thickening of the retina located less than 0.5 mm from the centre of the macula.
· Exudates (with thickening of adjacent retina) located less than 0.5 mm from the centre of the macula.
· An area of retinal thickening 1 disc diameter in size located less than 1 disc diameter from the centre of the macula.

For practical purposes, sight-threatening maculopathy is any retinopathy lesion within ½ a disc diameter of the centre of the macula; this simplified definition will assist the non-ophthalmologist in identifying what may be sight-threatening but this would not necessarily be an indication for laser treatment.

PRE-PROLIFERATIVE DIABETIC RETINOPATHY

Although classified as a subcategory of background retinopathy, pre-proliferative retinopathy is a sight-threatening condition that is usually considered separately from background disease. It also differs from background retinopathy in having four new features, i.e. cotton wool spots, retinal venous abnormalities, large blot intraretinal haemorrhages and intraretinal microvascular abnormalities.

Cotton wool spots

Cotton wool spots appear as pale cream patches of variable sizes (**Fig. 10.3**). They do not have clearly defined outlines and are most frequently seen in the posterior pole. A cotton wool spot is an area of infarction in the nerve fibre layer, and the appearance is due to swollen nerve axons with impaired axoplasmic flow. It therefore represents an area of localized retinal ischaemia and suggests the presence of arteriolar occlusion. Cotton wool spots persist for a long time, ranging from 8 to 17 months. Five or more cotton wool spots are generally required to suggest preproliferative disease.

Intraretinal microvascular abnormalities (IRMA)

These usually appear as irregular loops of vessels within the retina which may straddle normal vessels (**Fig. 10.3**). IRMA occur adjacent to areas of capillary bed closure and their origin is unclear. Unlike 'new vessels', IRMA do not always leak fluorescein, although some leakage may occur at their growing tips. At least two different theories exist as to what abnormal vasculature are presently classified as IRMA: shunt vessels and intraretinal new vessels.

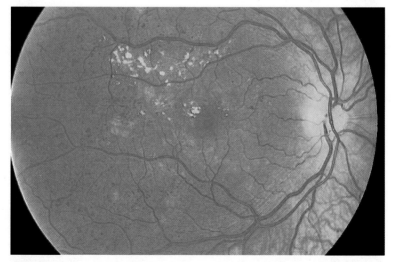

Fig. 10.3 Early preproliferative retinopathy with intraretinal microvascular abnormalities associated with cotton wool spots.

Venous abnormalities

Various abnormalities occur in the retinal veins in response to the hypoxic environment (**Fig. 10.4**). These take the form of:

- beading, e.g. the 'string-of-sausages' appearance;
- reduplication of veins, whereby the vein appears to divide into two parallel channels over a short segment; and
- venous loops, where the vein makes a sudden deviation in the form of a loop.

Venous abnormalities, particularly those of beading and reduplication, are strong indicators of hypoxia and suggest that new vessel development is imminent.

Deep retinal haemorrhages

These are large dark haemorrhages within the retina representing haemorrhagic infarction secondary to retinal arteriolar occlusion.

Proliferative diabetic retinopathy

Ischaemia within the retina due to widespread closure of capillary beds leads to newly formed blood vessels appearing on the retinal surface, or overlying the optic disc. These vessels extend in the plane between the retina and the vitreous and are accompanied by a supporting network of fibroglial proliferation.

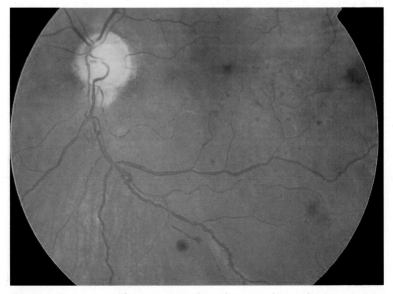

Fig. 10.4 Severe preproliferative retinopathy with venous abnormalities.

New vessels developing from the vasculature of the optic disc are called 'disc new vessels' (NVD) (**Fig. 10.5**) whilst those developing on the surface of the retina are called 'new vessels elsewhere' (NVE) (**Fig. 10.6**). It is thought that NVD represents severe generalized ischaemia of the retina, whereas NVE is a response to local ischaemia in the quadrant of the retina where they occur.

New vessels usually arise from a vein and have a haphazard growth pattern. As they grow, the combination of new vessels and supporting fibroglial tissue becomes adherent to both the retinal and posterior vitreous surfaces, inducing the vitreous to detach from the retina. The subsequent traction may cause haemorrhage either because the fragile new vessels break or because they are avulsed from their point of origin on the main retinal vessel. If bleeding is confined to the space between the retina and the vitreous, a preretinal or retro-hyaloid haemorrhage is clearly visible on ophthalmoscopy (the so-called 'boat shaped' haemorrhage with a fluid level appearance). Depending on whether the haemorrhage obscures the macula, vision may be severely affected or minimally compromised. If the haemorrhage is to break through into the main body of the vitreous, the view of the retina may be variably obscured, likewise the patient's vision. At worse, no view may be possible of the retina.

The second outcome of neovascular traction is a retinal detachment. A tractional retinal detachment usually occurs slowly, and may remain stable for years assuming laser treatment has been applied to control the neovascular process. A tractional retinal detachment affects vision in two ways. First, if it directly affects the fovea, vision will be reduced; if extrafoveal traction

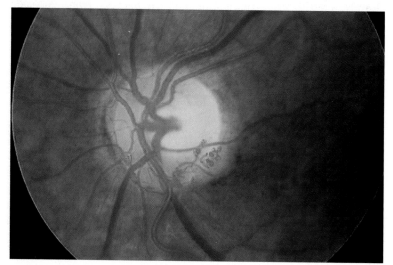

Fig. 10.5 Proliferative retinopathy with disc new vessels (NVD).

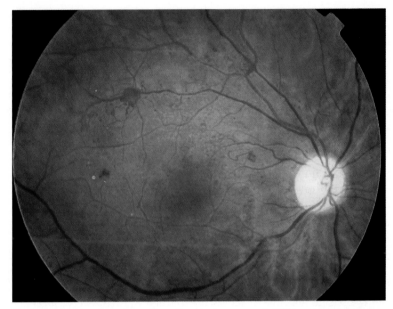

Fig. 10.6 Proliferative retinopathy with retinal new vessels (NVE).

exists, tension-induced retinal folds may secondarily affect the fovea, producing visual distortion. Secondly, a stable tractional detachment may suddenly become unstable if a full-thickness hole occurs in the retina, leading to
a rhegmatogenous retinal detachment which may spread to involve the fovea.

The proliferative process may not be confined to the posterior segment of
the eye. Iris neovascularization is a feared complication because of the risk of
neovascular or thrombotic glaucoma, a form of glaucoma which is difficult to
manage once established. As with retinal neovascularization, fibrous tissue
eventually develops which can occlude the trabecular meshwork and the
anterior chamber angle leading to uncontrolled neovascular glaucoma or secondary angle closure glaucoma, resulting in a painful, red blind eye.

DIAGNOSIS OF DIABETIC RETINOPATHY

It is essential to examine patients with diabetes regularly to screen for the
presence of symptomless retinopathy. Retinopathy screening is presently performed by healthcare professionals in a variety of disciplines, including
optometrists, nurses, medical photographers, general practitioners and diabetologists using a variety of techniques, e.g. direct and indirect ophthalmoscopy and retinal photography.

Screening for diabetic retinopathy

Diabetic retinopathy is a disease which fulfills all the necessary criteria for a screening programme. Those at risk form an identifiable population, it has a recognized disease pattern and laser treatment, if performed early, is effective in preventing loss of vision, particularly in proliferative disease. Advanced disease, when diagnosed late, is less amenable to treatment and much more costly, both economically and in terms of the patient's quality of life.

In the UK and many other countries, however, there is no national strategy for the screening of diabetic retinopathy. In any one year in the UK, the proportion of diabetic patients who receive retinopathy screening varies from 38% to 85%, and from 14% to 97% between different primary care practices. Approximately 10% of specialist diabetes units in England and Wales do not have a systematic screening service; among the 90% that do, the proportion of patients screened varies from 25% to >95%.

A variety of local methods are in use in the UK, e.g. selected optometrists accredited to perform the screening using slit-lamp biomicroscopy, and schemes that are based on retinal photography, either fixed-site or via a mobile unit.

Techniques for screening

Direct ophthalmoscopy using a hand-held ophthalmoscope is used to a varying extent, and with varying degrees of success, by general practitioners, optometrists and diabetologists. It is technically difficult, allowing only a two-dimensional view of the retina (therefore retinal oedema cannot be accurately diagnosed using this technique). The peripheral parts of the retina are difficult to examine using this technique. It is a form of examination that has largely been abandoned by ophthalmologists, who now mainly examine the retina by slit-lamp biomicroscopy.

Slit-lamp biomicroscopy provides a much wider three-dimensional view of the retina using a 78 or 90 dioptre lens. Although an effective technique, it is very skill-dependent and the operator requires extensive training. Both methods of ophthalmoscopy have to be performed with mydriasis (dilated pupils) and both have the disadvantage of not providing a hard record for qualitative assessment and for monitoring signs of progression of disease.

Retinal photography is a technique that is more easily acquired, and the image can be interpreted later by another health professional, e.g. diabetologist, ophthalmologist or a specially trained grader. The number of ungradeable photographs ranges from 3.7% to 20%, the failure rate being lower with mydriasis. Increasingly, digital photography is supplanting the analogue techniques of slides and Polaroid photography. It has major advantages in its ease of image acquisition, data storage and there is also the option of electronic data transfer. The computerized interpretation of images is a real possibility and the screening process may eventually become entirely electronic.

The British Diabetic Association (BDA) has proposed that a screening test for diabetic retinopathy should have at least 80% sensitivity and 95% specificity. In a wide ranging review of multiple studies examining the effectiveness of direct ophthalmoscopy, indirect ophthalmoscopy and retinal photography, it has been reported that retinal photography with a dilated pupil is the most effective. Most of the studies that employed retinal photography had sensitivity levels of over 80%, and mydriatic photographs gave an even higher level of sensitivity.

Proposed UK national screening scheme

Screening for retinopathy in the UK is likely to change as part of the 'Preservation of sight in diabetes: a risk reduction programme' initiative. A nationwide screening programme will be established by 2005/2006 with clear aims: (1) to reduce the rate of avoidable visual loss by early detection of sight-threatening retinopathy so that it can be treated promptly; and (2) the detection of any retinopathy, so that the diabetic patient can be made aware that changes have begun to occur in their eyes, and attempts can be made to improve glycaemic and blood pressure control.

The main features of this screening program would include:

- Target population: all diabetic patients, types 1 and 2, over 12 years of age, or postpuberty; a database needs to be established probably through a centralized screening office collaborating with general practitioners.
- Frequency: annually initially but after a few screening rounds those deemed to be at low risk can then be screened less frequently.
- Technique: mydriatic digital photography (two fields, macular and nasal) with visual acuity measurement (visual acuity alone will not lead to referral to an assessment clinic unless accompanied by retinopathy, although the general practitioner will be informed if visual acuity falls below 6/12 in either eye). It is still unclear who will be taking the photographs and it may be up to individual health districts to decide whether to employ specific photographers or to pay local optometrists to perform the task.
- Examination: grading of photographs by specially trained graders using a standardized grading scheme employing reference images, with opinions from ophthalmologists and/or diabetologists if required.
- Positive patients: referral to special assessment clinics at convenient ophthalmology departments.

CURRENT ISSUES

· The classification of diabetic retinopathy into background and proliferative stages is well established and assists in the management of sight-threatening retinopathy.
· Screening for diabetic retinopathy in many countries, including the UK, is not sufficiently well established or co-ordinated to achieve the standards required by the St Vincent declaration of 1989.
· The most sensitive screening technique for diabetic retinopathy is mydriatic fundus photography and the least effective is direct ophthalmoscopy.
· Successful retinopathy screening is principally technique-dependent and less personnel-dependent.

FURTHER READING

Bachmann MO, Nelson SJ. Impact of diabetic retinopathy screening on a British district population: case detection and blindness prevention in an evidence-based model. *J Epidemiol Community Health* 1998; **52**: 45–52.

Bagga P, Verma D, Walton C, Masson EA, Hepburn DA. Survey of diabetic retinopathy screening services in England and Wales. *Diabetic Medicine* 1998; **15**: 780–2.

Garvican L, Clowes J, Gillow T. Preservation of sight in diabetes: developing a national risk reduction programme. *Diabetic Medicine* 2000; **17**: 627–34.

Hart PM, Harding S. Is it time for a national screening programme for sight threatening retinopathy? *Eye* 1999; **13**: 129–30.

Hutchinson A, McIntosh A, Peters J *et al.* Effectiveness of screening and monitoring tests for diabetic retinopathy—a systematic review. *Diabetic Medicine* 2000; **17**: 495–506.

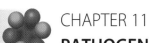

CHAPTER 11
PATHOGENESIS OF DIABETIC RETINOPATHY

INTRODUCTION

There are multiple pathophysiological mechanisms in diabetic retinopathy that combine to produce its two defining features, both of which occur in the retinal vasculature. First, there is increased vascular permeability due to a breakdown in the blood–retinal barrier, which results in vascular leakage and the accumulation of extracellular fluid. The second pathological process is the occlusion of capillary beds giving rise to retinal ischaemia, which leads eventually to the development of new vessels. Both of these key pathological features coexist, and are responsible for the visual problems of background retinopathy and proliferative retinopathy, respectively.

These two pathological processes are reflected at the microscopic level by characteristic abnormalities:

- A thickened capillary basement membrane which results in:
  - Impaired ability of the basement membrane to bind and inactivate various molecules, in part due to a reduction in heparan sulphate proteoglycan.
  - Reduced endothelial cell–pericyte contact, which reduces the normal inhibitory effect of pericytes on endothelial cell proliferation.
  - The thickened basement membrane becomes less pliable and restricts capillary motion.
- Loss of capillary pericytes leads to weak areas in the capillary wall and formation of microaneurysms with subsequent vascular leakage. Pericytes also inhibit the proliferation of endothelial cells and their early loss may contribute towards the neovascularization process.
- Loss of capillary endothelial cells. Acellular capillaries are non-functional, devoid of blood and therefore lead to retinal hypoxia.

Several biochemical mechanisms have been identified which may independently or in combination produce the morphological, structural and functional abnormalities characteristic of diabetic retinopathy.

THE POLYOL PATHWAY

Glucose is metabolized via the polyol pathway when other metabolic pathways are saturated, i.e. it is only important in the presence of hyperglycaemia. This is because the principal enzyme in the pathway, aldose reductase, has a low affinity for glucose. Aldose reductase, which is present in all tissues affected by diabetic microangiopathy, converts glucose into sorbitol (**Fig. 11.1**). Sorbitol is then metabolized into fructose by sorbitol dehydrogenase, but this reaction is much slower than that of aldose reductase. The net result is an accumulation of sor-

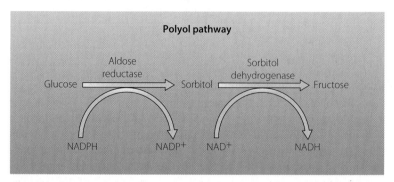

Fig. 11.1 Glucose is metabolized by aldose reductase to sorbitol and subsequently to fructose via the polyol pathway.

bitol which crosses the cell membrane very slowly; the resulting high intracellular concentration of sorbitol increases osmotic pressure and draws water into the cell. This causes intracellular oedema which may disrupt cell function.

The polyol pathway was first implicated as a pathogenic mechanism in rats fed a high galactose diet, which causes diabetic retinopathy-like lesions; however, if the animals were simultaneously fed an aldose reductase inhibitor these lesions did not develop.

Increased aldose reductase activity may also mediate cellular damage through other mechanisms in addition to the effect on osmotic pressure (**Fig. 11.2**). For example, the polyol pathway consumes reduced nicotinamide adenine dinucleotide phosphate (NADPH) and thus impairs the free-radical scavenging ability. The polyol pathway also reduces intracellular levels of myoinositol, which is required for Na^+/K^+-ATPase activity. This is a ubiquitous enzyme, being part of the cell membrane Na^+ pump, and is an essential component affecting cell functions as diverse as contractility, differentiation and growth. Myoinositol also competes with glucose to cross cell membranes and therefore its uptake is also reduced by hyperglycaemia.

Activation of the polyol pathway may be responsible for the thickened capillary basement membrane. There is also some evidence indicating that the sorbitol pathway is present in pericytes, but not endothelial cells, and that this may account for the early preferential loss of capillary pericytes.

ACTIVATION OF PROTEIN KINASE C

Another biochemical pathway affected by hyperglycaemia is the increased activity of protein kinase C (PKC). PKC is up-regulated by hyperglycaemia, with the effect persistent for a considerable period (weeks) after normalization of blood glucose. Glucose metabolized through the glycolytic pathway

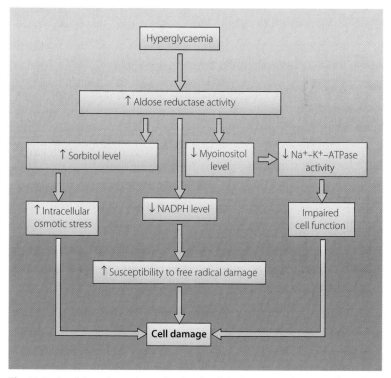

Fig. 11.2 Possible pathogenic mechanism for diabetic retinopathy arising from the polyol pathway.

generates diacylglycerol as a by-product, which in turn activates PKC. This reaction can be further potentiated by altered intracellular redox potential, e.g. via reduced intracellular NADPH (through increased consumption in the polyol pathway), and oxidants such as hydrogen peroxide can synergistically enhance PKC activation.

PKC is widely distributed and acts as an intracellular signal transducer for many cytokines and hormones acting upon a cell; it is an important mediator of various cell functions including growth and differentiation, vascular permeability, DNA synthesis, basement membrane turnover and vascular smooth muscle contraction.

Increased PKC activity, especially the PKC-β isoform, has been implicated in the pathogenesis of diabetic retinopathy in the following ways:
- Basement membrane thickening, probably through increasing synthesis of collagen and fibronectin.
- Retinal vasoconstriction, in part via inhibition of nitric oxide-mediated

vasodilation and increased endothelin-1 expression, thus altering retinal blood flow.

- Increased vascular permeability by phosphorylating and inactivating intercellular proteins normally responsible for tight-junctions.
- Increased production of vascular permeability factor (VPF) in response to high glucose. Additionally, the action of VPF on endothelial cells, i.e. both its mitogenic and permeability-inducing actions, have in turn been shown to be mediated by PKC.
- Increased endothelial surface expression of adhesion molecules such as intercellular adhesions molecule-1 (ICAM-1), thereby increasing cellular adhesion to circulating platelets.
- Decreased Na^+/K^+-ATPase activity, potentiating any similar effect by increased polyol pathway activity. This enzyme is an important component of the retinal pigment epithelium pump's ability to remove extracellular fluid.

A selective PKC-β inhibitor, LY333531 (a bisindoylmaleimide) has been found to reverse or prevent several of the dysfunctions described above, including normalization of retinal haemodynamics and inhibition of retinal neovascularization. Clinical trials using this promising compound are ongoing. Vitamin E has also been shown to ameliorate PKC activation by decreasing diacylglycerol levels.

NON-ENZYMATIC GLYCATION OF PROTEINS

Glucose molecules are able to attach onto lysine residues of proteins (Maillard reaction), both extracellularly and intracellularly; the rate at which this occurs depends upon the ambient glucose concentration and duration of exposure. Proteins affected by this process include haemoglobin (producing glycosylated haemoglobin that is employed as an indicator of recent glycaemic control), cell membrane proteins, lens crystallins, plasma proteins and collagen. The initial product is reversible, but it eventually transforms into a more stable product (Amadori rearrangement) which is still potentially but slowly reversible. These early glycation products affect cell function, including regulation of free radical-mediated vascular damage and uptake of low-density lipoproteins (LDL). The early glycation products may break-down but long-lived proteins, such as collagen, may evolve through further irreversible rearrangements (covalent bonding), forming advanced glycosylation end-products (AGE).

Many cell types, including pericytes, endothelial cells, smooth muscle cells, lymphocytes and monocytes, possess surface receptors for AGE. The binding of AGE to receptors on cells (termed RAGE to mean 'receptor for AGE') may lead to: (1) increased production of cytokines and surface adhesion molecules; (2) increased vascular permeability and changes in cellular proliferation; (3) up-regulation of extracellular matrix gene expression leading to increased production of basement membrane components; and (4) toxicity to retinal capillary pericytes with mitogenic stimulation of endothelial cells.

Aminoguanidine is an inhibitor of this glycation process, and in diabetic animals produces a reduction in the severity of diabetic retinopathy. There is recent evidence, however, that the beneficial effect of aminoguanidine on diabetic retinopathy may not be solely due to its effect on AGE; in diabetic rats, aminoguanidine was found to reduce early apoptosis of retinal microvascular cells independently of any reduction in glycosylated protein products. Aminoguanidine has also been shown to normalize several hyperglycaemia-induced features in experimental animals such as oxidative stress and augmented PKC activity.

HAEMORHEOLOGICAL FACTORS

Haemorheological factors implicated in the pathogenesis of diabetic retinopathy include increased blood viscosity, increased platelet aggregation, increased leucocyte adhesion and decreased red cell deformability. Blood viscosity is increased in diabetic patients, particularly those with proliferative retinopathy, due to increased plasma proteins and decreased red cell deformability.

Increased platelet aggregation, delayed platelet disaggregation and increased platelet-derived thromboxane B_2 have all been reported in diabetic patients, all of which contribute towards a procoagulant state. Drugs that inhibit platelet aggregation, however, have little or no effect on the progression of diabetic retinopathy.

There is increasing interest in the role that leucocytes may play in the development of capillary occlusion. They are large cells with a rigid cytoplasmic structure and a natural tendency to adhere onto vascular endothelium. They also have the capacity to generate toxic superoxide radicals and proteolytic enzymes. Plugs of leucocytes have been found in the lumen of occluded capillaries.

ABNORMAL RETINAL BLOOD FLOW

Poor glycaemic control increases microvascular blood flow in several tissues including the retina, and various mechanisms have been proposed (**Fig. 11.3**). Retinal glucose is metabolized mainly through the glycolytic pathway and in hyperglycaemic conditions this can lead to an accumulation of retinal lactate which mimics a hypoxic environment leading to an autoregulatory hyperperfusion. A similar effect occurs via the polyol pathway when an imbalance in the ratio of NAD^+ to NADH mimics a hypoxic environment. Thus, pseudohypoxia may affect microvascular haemodynamics resulting in increased retinal blood flow. In the presence of capillary occlusion, true hypoxia exists which leads to increased blood flow, through autoregulatory mechanisms, in capillary beds which are still perfused.

Increased retinal blood flow may inflict damage upon the retinal vasculature in a number of ways:

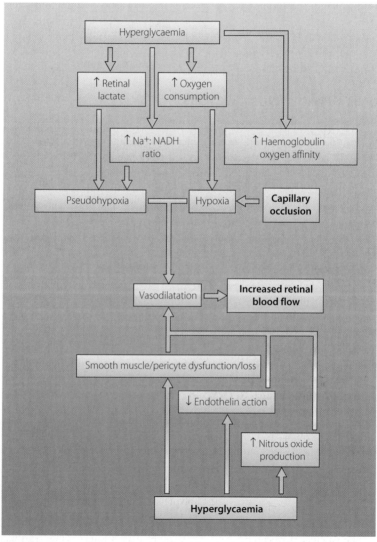

Fig. 11.3 Causes of increased retinal blood flow in diabetic retinopathy.

- Increased 'shear stress' upon the vascular endothelium may increase its permeability to macromolecules and, if the forces are sufficiently high, cause direct morphological changes.
- The regulatory, protective mechanisms of the retinal microcirculation may be compromised by early compensatory changes, such as a thickened basement membrane.
- Flow-induced vessel dilatation leads to vascular stretching and to a breakdown of the blood–retinal barrier.
- Increased blood flow compounds the hyperpermeable state of the retinal vessels.

GLUCOSE-INDUCED APOPTOSIS

There is evidence that high circulating glucose concentrations can paradoxically lead to a low pericyte glucose concentration; a high glucose level decreases the glucose transport activity in pericytes but not endothelial cells. Pericytes undergo apoptosis if the glucose level is suddenly reduced; this mimics the situation in diabetic patients where the blood glucose level can fluctuate quite significantly. Apoptosis of endothelial cells has also been demonstrated in high glucose concentrations.

GROWTH FACTORS

The normal human retina has a very stable vascular endothelial cell population with minimal mitotic activity. However, when a hypoxic environment exists following extensive closure of capillary beds, it has been postulated, firstly by Michaelson in 1948, that a diffusible angiogenic factor(s) is produced which leads to the development of the new blood vessels seen in proliferative retinopathy. Various agents which may fulfil this role have been identified and they include:

- Basic fibroblast growth factor (bFGF); levels are increased in the vitreous from eyes with active proliferative retinopathy and its release has been associated with cell damage or death.
- Insulin-like growth factor 1 (IGF-1), which is mainly produced by the liver but also produced by retinal endothelial cells. It has been shown to stimulate endothelial cell growth and retinal vascular permeability.
- Transforming growth factor β (TGFβ) is responsible for the normal inhibitory effect exerted by pericytes on endothelial cell division, but it also plays a role in the later stages of angiogenesis.
- Vascular permeability factor (VPF) is probably the most important growth factor. It modulates angiogenesis, promotes endothelial cell proliferation and vascular permeability, and increases the expression of ICAM-1. It has also been demonstrated to lead to endothelial cell hypertrophy which has

been postulated to play a role in capillary closure. VPF is up-regulated by glucose and hypoxia.

Vascular permeability factor (also known as vascular endothelial growth factor, VEGF)

Even diabetic eyes with no overt signs of retinopathy have higher levels of VPF compared with normal eyes, suggesting that VPF is important in the early stages of retinopathy when it may induce increased vascular permeability. VPF is 50 000 times more potent than histamine in promoting vascular leakage and it may influence the phenotype of the capillary endothelium, for example from non-fenestrated to fenestrated.

High-affinity, membrane-bound VPF receptors have been identified on both retinal endothelial cells and retinal pigment epithelial cells. Many retinal cell lines are capable of producing VPF. VPF injected into the vitreous of primates has produced lesions consistent with background and preproliferative retinopathy, but other factors may be required for VPF to produce neovascularization.

CURRENT ISSUES

- Aminoguanidine, an inhibitor of AGE formation, has been found to ameliorate retinopathy in animal models although its effect may not be solely on AGE formation, for example there is some evidence to suggest it affects VPF production and PKC activity.
- Leukocytes have been implicated in vascular leakage and capillary closure because of their large size, increased adhesiveness to vascular endothelium, reduced deformability in diabetes, and their ability to release toxic superoxide radicals and enzymes when activated.
- VPF is probably the most important of the growth factors implicated in the pathogenesis of diabetic retinopathy. The retina produces VPF and receptors for VPF exist on retinal endothelial cells as well as retinal pigment epithelial cells. VPF activity in the eye is increased by hyperglycaemia and hypoxia. VPF promotes vascular leakage and neovascularization, and is therefore implicated in both of the principal features of diabetic retinopathy.
- PKC is up-regulated by hyperglycaemia and its activity is closely linked with that of VPF. PKC mediates VPF formation and VPF action.

FURTHER READING

Aiello LP, Bursell SE, Clermont A *et al.* Vascular endothelial growth factor-induced retinal permeability is mediated by protein kinase C *in vivo* and suppressed by an orally effective beta-isoform-selective inhibitor. *Diabetes* 1997; **46**: 1473–80.

Ferrara N. Vascular endothelial growth factor. The trigger for neovascularization in the eye. *Laboratory Invest* 1995; **72**: 615–18.

Meier M, King GL. Protein kinase C activation and its pharmacological inhibition in vascular disease. *Vascular Medicine* 2000; **5**: 173–185.

Miyamoto K, Ogura Y. Pathogenetic potential of leucocytes in diabetic retinopathy. *Semin Ophthalmol* 1999; **14**: 233–239.

Ozaki H, Seo MS, Ozaki K, Yamada H, Yamada E, Okamoto N, Hofmann F, Wood JM, Campochiaro PA. Blockade of vascular endothelial cell growth factor receptor signalling is sufficient to completely prevent retinal neovascularization. *Am J Pathol* 2000; **156**: 697–707.

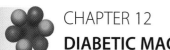

CHAPTER 12
DIABETIC MACULOPATHY

Hean-Choon Chen FRCS, FRCOpath   119

INTRODUCTION

Diabetic maculopathy is the commonest cause of visual loss in patients with diabetes and it can be defined as the presence of sight-threatening lesions within the macula. These lesions commonly consist of microaneurysms, haemorrhages and exudates. The cause of visual loss is a consequence of either or both of the following:

- leaking blood vessels leading to exudate formation, accumulation of extra-cellular fluid and macular oedema (exudative diabetic maculopathy or diabetic macular oedema); and
- capillary closure giving rise to macular ischaemia (ischaemic diabetic maculopathy).

Loss of vision from exudation and oedema is the commoner of the two mechanisms and is fortunately responsive to laser treatment, at least in part. There is no treatment for macular ischaemia.

EPIDEMIOLOGY

The Wisconsin Epidemiologic Study of Diabetic Retinopathy (WESDR) reported an overall prevalence rate of 10% for macular oedema; predictably, the prevalence increases with increasing severity of overall retinopathy status, ranging from approximately 2% in those with mild background retinopathy to 20–37% in those with moderate to severe background disease, and in those with proliferative retinopathy the prevalence of macular oedema was approximately 70% (**Table 12.1**). The prevalence of maculopathy also increases with duration of diabetes, and is higher in type 2 compared with type 1 diabetes (**Figs 12.1 and 12.2**).

DEFINITIONS

Exudative maculopathy
The Early Treatment Diabetic Retinopathy Study (ETDRS) group produced a list of criteria to denote clinically significant macular oedema, i.e. maculopathy for which laser treatment is indicated (see Chapter 10).

Ischaemic maculopathy
The normal fovea possesses a central avascular area known as the foveolar avascular zone (FAZ); this exists so as to provide the centre of the fovea with the least possible impedance to incident light. In the normal eye, the FAZ

Diabetes-related activation of DAG-PKC pathway in vascular cells and tissues								
	Younger onset			Older onset				
	Duration 10+ years			Duration 0–14 years			Duration 15+ years	
Retinopathy status	No.	% Macular oedema	P	No.	% Macular oedema	P	No.	% Macular oedema	P
Non-proliferative								
Mild	172	1.7	–	152	2.6	–	126	6.3	–
Moderate to severe	128	20.3	<0.001	60	36.7	<0.001	87	63.2	<0.001
Proliferative	85	69.7	–	26	73.1	–	35	74.3	

*Percentage with macular oedema = (number of persons with macular oedema status 2 or 3 in either or both eyes/number of persons with macular oedema status 0 in both eyes + number of persons with macular oedema status 2 or 3 in either or both eyes) × 100.

Table 12.1   Relationship of diabetic retinopathy with macular oedema* and duration of diabetes (Wisconsin, HAS-1, 1980–82). The Wisconsin Epidemiologic Study of Diabetic Retinopathy. IV. Diabetic macular oedema. *Ophthalmology* 1984; **91:** 1464–74.

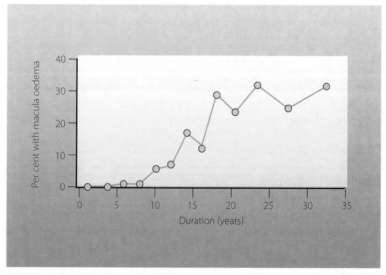

Fig. 12.1   Frequency of macular oedema by duration of diabetes in years for insulin-taking early onset persons. *Ophthalmology* 1984; **91:** 1464–74.

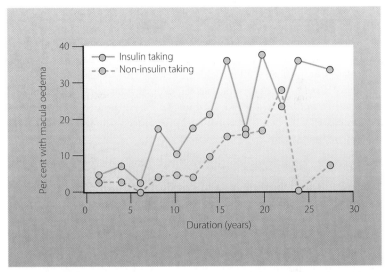

Fig. 12.2 Frequency of macular oedema by duration of diabetes for insulin- and non-insulin-taking older onset persons. The Wisconsin Epidemiologic Study of Diabetic Retinopathy. IV. Diabetic macular oedema. *Ophthalmology* 1984; **91**: 1464–74.

varies significantly in size with an average of approximately 0.5–0.6 mm. In ischaemic maculopathy, there is a gradual increase in the size of FAZ. Although there is no defining measurement of FAZ for a diagnosis of ischaemic maculopathy, when the diameter of FAZ exceeds 1 mm vision is usually compromised (**Fig. 12.3**).

DIAGNOSIS

The diagnosis of diabetic maculopathy is made clinically and, when necessary, with the aid of fluorescein angiography. The following changes in visual function may raise the suspicion of macular disease:

· reduced visual acuity;
· reduced contrast sensitivity; and
· colour vision defects, usually along the blue-yellow (tritan-like) axis, may occur from an early stage in the disease and may even predate clinically visible lesions.

Clinically, the presence of microaneurysms and exudates indicates the presence of pathological vascular leakage, although these changes alone may not reduce visual acuity. The retinal pigment epithelial 'pump' and surrounding competent capillaries are able to remove extravasated fluid and extracellular fluid accumulates when the rate of leakage exceeds the capacity for fluid removal, giving rise to retinal thickening. Vision is affected when this occurs at the centre of the macula. However, exudates in large numbers, and especially at the centre of the macula, can also affect vision in the absence of retinal thickening (probably due to direct photoreceptor damage). When large numbers of exudates are present, macular oedema is usually also present. It is not unusual to observe a paradoxical increase in the number of exudates as oedema dissipates, since lipoproteins are precipitated within the retina as the water component of oedema is removed.

The diagnosis of macular thickening requires stereoscopic views of the macula. This is possible with slit-lamp biomicroscopy using either a non-contact 78 or 90 dioptre lens, or with a fundus contact lens. The contact lenses provide better stereopsis and may be better at detecting subtle degrees of retinal thickening. Fluorescein angiography is usually not necessary in the diagnosis of macular oedema. However, when there is an unexplained loss of vision, i.e. when it cannot be attributed to vascular leakage, fluorescein angiography is helpful. The diagnosis of macular ischaemia can only be definitively made with fluorescein angiography.

Fluorescein angiography

Fluorescein angiography outlines the retinal circulation, illuminating the otherwise invisible microvasculature. It is a photographic investigation technique that uses an adapted fundus camera. Fluorescein, a vegetable dye extract, is able to absorb light with a wavelength of approximately 490 nm (blue light) and in response emits light at a longer wavelength of 530 nm (green light). Fluorescein is injected into an antecubital vein (usually 5 ml of

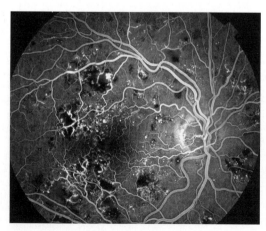

Fig. 12.3 This fluorescein angiogram of the posterior pole of the eye demonstrates the presence of ischaemic maculopathy with an enlarged foveal avascular zone.

a 10% solution), where it becomes 70–85% plasma-protein bound, and photographs are taken of the fundus as it traverses the retinal circulation. The adapted fundus camera possesses two filters to ensure that blue light enters the eye and yellow-green light enters the camera, where it is captured on film. Photographs are usually taken from about 10 seconds after injection and thereafter at 1–2-second intervals. Late pictures may be taken after a few minutes to determine the possible presence of late leakage.

Fluorescein angiography provides assistance in the diagnosis of:

- Capillary closure or non-perfusion, especially in the macula, where capillaries exist as a monolayer with an increased melanin background, providing greater contrast. This is particularly helpful in the diagnosis of ischaemic maculopathy, where, in good quality fluorescein angiographic pictures, FAZ is clearly delineated.
- Vascular leakage, although fluorescein angiography is seldom required to make this diagnosis (**Fig. 12.4**). Cystoid macular oedema takes on a characteristic petalloid appearance (**Fig. 12.5**).
- Subtle neovascularization, which may not be immediately obvious on clinical examination; new vessels do not possess a normal blood–retinal barrier (BRB) and are hyperpermeable, therefore giving rise to extensive fluorescein leakage. Several other retinopathy lesions can also be highlighted, e.g. microaneurysms and intraretinal neovascular abnormalities (IRMA).

PATHOGENESIS

Exudative maculopathy or macular oedema is the consequence of a breakdown of the BRB, more specifically the inner BRB, i.e. the retinal capillary endothelium. This is usually at sites of microaneurysms although other

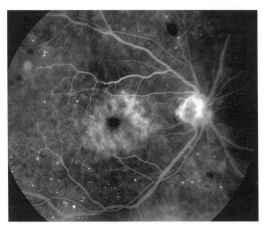

Fig. 12.4 Fluorescein angiogram demonstrating diffuse macular leakage.

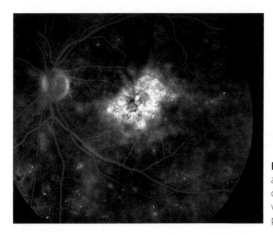

Fig. 12.5 Fluorescein angiogram demonstrating cystoid macular oedema with its characteristic petal-like leakage pattern.

retinopathy lesions also signify breaches in the BRB such as dilated capillaries, IRMA and retinal neovascularization.

There is, however, also some evidence suggesting a breakdown in the outer BRB, i.e. the retinal pigment epithelium (RPE), as well. The RPE forms a barrier between the neural retina and the choriocapillaris, the capillary network of the choroid, which is highly permeable to macromolecules (unlike retinal capillaries). The normally tight junctions of the RPE therefore maintain a diffusion gradient for water from retina to choroid because of the higher oncotic pressure within the choroid.

It has also recently been demonstrated that a taut, thickened posterior hyaloid (vitreous), which is still attached to the retina, can give rise to traction upon the macula producing intraretinal cystic spaces, and possibly a tractional detachment. These changes in the posterior hyaloid usually occur in response to ischaemic disease and therefore this form of macular oedema more frequently occurs in severe forms of retinopathy.

TREATMENT

Ischaemic maculopathy is not amenable to treatment. Exudative maculopathy may, for treatment purposes, be subclassified into two varieties:

- Focal oedema. This is a localized area of leakage, usually from a cluster of microaneurysms which exist in the centre of an area of oedema. The area affected is usually circular and its periphery often delineated by a ring of exudates, the so-called 'circinate of exudates'.
- Diffuse oedema. Leakage appears to occur from a large area of dilated capillaries, sometimes with little evidence of exudate formation. This is

possibly due to capillary beds dilating to compensate for surrounding areas of capillary occlusion, or there may be an autoregulatory increase in local retinal blood flow. Prolonged diffuse oedema can lead to the formation of cystic spaces in the centre of the macula, known as cystoid macular oedema (CMO), and is more likely to be associated with systemic problems such as renal failure and uncontrolled hypertension.

Both forms of oedema can coexist. There will usually be areas of focal leakage in patients with diffuse oedema but an area of focal oedema frequently exists in isolation. The visual deficit is usually more severe in cases of diffuse oedema, which is unfortunately also more refractory to treatment, particularly in the presence of cystoid oedema.

Laser therapy

Laser therapy is effective in both focal and diffuse macular oedema. In focal oedema, the treatment is applied directly at the area(s) of leakage, for example the microaneurysms at the centre of a ring of exudates. An attempt may be made to coagulate the microaneurysm. The ETDRS protocol included direct treatment of microaneurysms greater than 40 µm in diameter. The technique employed to do this is to initially 'whiten' the underlying retinal pigment epithelium using a 100-µm spot size. The aim of this step is to ensure that the whitened underlying tissue will no longer absorb the energy from subsequent laser shots. The spot size should then be reduced to 50 µm and aimed at the microaneurysm, with the aim of turning it white or a darker shade of red.

In diffuse oedema the method used is known as 'grid macular treatment'. It involves applying laser burns with a spot size of between 100 µm and 200 µm, aiming for a blanching effect of the retinal pigment epithelium, i.e. a grey-white effect. The spots are applied to cover the part of the macula that is thickened, sparing the fovea; treatment should commence approximately 500 µm from the centre of the macula and be spaced about one burn-width apart. If oedema persists, retreatment with laser burns applied closer to the centre of the macula can be applied; the ETDRS protocol allowed for treatment from 300 µm from the centre of the macula, unless there is perifoveal capillary dropout. Treatment over the papillo-macular bundle is possible since the nerve fibre layer is spared, as the level of laser energy used affects only the pigment epithelium and its immediate neighbours. The ETDRS protocol advocated treating not just the areas that were oedematous but also any adjacent areas of capillary non-perfusion.

Treatment should be applied using an appropriate contact lens to provide good visibility of the macula, e.g. the wide-angle Volk Transequator. The type of thermal laser wavelength used should be either green (e.g. argon and double-frequency YAG lasers) or yellow (dye laser); blue light laser should be avoided in treatment of the macula because the absorption of blue light by abundant macular xanthophyll pigment can cause greater degrees of collateral damage to the retina. The red light of the krypton laser will not be absorbed by haemoglobin and therefore will not be useful in closing microaneurysms.

At the commencement of treatment, it is prudent to assess the energy requirement away from areas close to the fovea, perhaps with a trial shot a short distance away. An initial energy setting of approximately 80–100 mW should be considered with a pulse duration of 0.1 seconds; these settings may then be modified according to the response.

Following treatment, an appropriate review interval will be between 2 and 4 months. It often takes this period of time for any effect on oedema resolution to become obvious.

Surgical procedures

If a taut posterior hyaloid is visible, pars plana vitrectomy has been found to be effective in resolving macular oedema. Features supporting this particular treatment option may include oedema resistant to grid laser treatment and the presence of cystoid oedema. Optical coherence tomography (OCT) may help in the identification of traction upon the macula but this form of investigation is not widely available. Vitrectomy may improve macular oedema even in the absence of signs suggesting vitreo-macular traction. Large subfoveal exudates may be removed surgically and this form of treatment has been reported with some success.

THE EFFECTIVENESS OF LASER TREATMENT

In treating focal leakage, successful closure of the leaking points, i.e. the microaneurysms, implies that leakage stops. However, part of the success is likely to be due to those factors which lead to the resolution of oedema following treatment for diffuse leakage.

Why laser treatment works in the treatment of diffuse leakage is unclear. Because the laser is targeted at the retinal pigment epithelium, the actual leaking points, i.e. the retinal capillaries, are not directly treated. Various hypotheses have been formulated to explain the therapeutic benefits of laser:

- Laser-damaged pigment epithelial cells regenerate and the new cells that fill the gaps created by thermal necrosis may create a more effective outer BRB.
- The laser also damages and causes loss of retinal photoreceptor cells, which are the major consumers of oxygen within the neural retina. This may relieve hypoxia and reduce the autoregulatory increment in blood flow through dilated capillary beds, thereby reducing leakage.

- The effect of the laser on the pigment epithelium may release a diffusible factor that induces retinal capillary repair, leading to a restoration of the inner BRB.

Laser treatment of diabetic maculopathy is not always successful; it is frequently only able to maintain current levels of vision, or slow the rate of progression, rather than lead to an improvement in vision.

If macular oedema coexists with a degree of ischaemia, it is reasonable to apply laser treatment although the prognosis is poorer compared with eyes without ischaemia. The diagnosis of ischaemia may be difficult in the presence of significant leakage since this obscures the view of the retinal microcirculation on fluorescein angiograms.

Complications of macular laser treatment

- Accidental damage to the foveola.
- Rupture of Bruch's membrane with use of high laser energy, which may lead to the formation of a choroidal neovascular membrane.
- Development of paracentral scotomata; these may be subtle and detectable only with more specialized perimetric techniques, such as blue-on-yellow perimetry.
- Submacular fibrosis from laser scars which appear to spread and merge.

WHEN SHOULD LASER TREATMENT BE APPLIED?

If clinically significant macular oedema (CSMO) exists, laser treatment should be applied soon, i.e. within weeks, and this is especially so if the centre of the macula is involved or directly threatened. When macular oedema coexists with proliferative retinopathy, the ETDRS group has clearly demonstrated that scatter photocoagulation leads to a worsening of the macular situation. It is recommended that whenever possible the macula should be treated first, or simultaneously, with the scatter treatment initially confined to the nasal quadrants.

Intraocular surgery, for example cataract extraction, has been shown to worsen maculopathy and, if the view allows it, macular laser treatment should be applied before the patient undergoes cataract surgery. If maculopathy is present but has not yet reached the severity of CSMO, the patient should be closely observed in the postoperative period as the level of maculopathy is very likely to increase in severity. A significant proportion of patients who develop macular oedema after cataract surgery will experience a spontaneous regression in their oedema, usually over several months after surgery, particularly if the underlying retinopathy status is mild. However, if oedema was present preoperatively, any worsening is likely to be persistent.

MICROPULSED DIODE LASER

This is a relatively novel approach using a diode laser with a wavelength of 810 nm (invisible, infrared wavelength) and the laser applied in a 'micropulse' fashion, i.e. frequent, short (microsecond) pulses delivering subthreshold laser energy (an energy level that does not produce an immediate, clinically evident effect). The energy is delivered in 'envelopes', each consisting of multiple short pulses. The advantage over conventional macular laser treatment is the specific targeting of the laser on the retinal pigment epithelium, therefore inducing less damage to surrounding tissues with fewer complications.

CURRENT DEVELOPMENT

- The ETDRS group has recommended laser treatment for those patients with features fulfilling the 'clinically significant macular oedema' criteria.
- Laser treatment is most likely to maintain current levels of vision, or retard the rate of progression of visual loss, rather than produce an improvement in vision.
- Laser treatment should be applied using a green or yellow wavelength, and may be applied in a focal and/or grid fashion for localized areas of leakage or diffuse leakage, respectively.
- Pars plana vitrectomy is effective in reducing diffuse macular oedema if a taut thickened posterior hyaloid is present. There is also evidence that persistent diabetic cystoid macular oedema may respond to pars plana vitrectomy, even if there is no clinical evidence of vitreous traction upon the macula.

FURTHER READING

Early Treatment Diabetic Retinopathy Study Research Group: Photocoagulation for diabetic macular oedema: Early Treatment Diabetic Retinopathy Study report number 1. *Arch Ophthalmol* 1985; **103**: 1796–1806.

Ikeda T, Sato K, Katano T, Hayashi Y. Vitrectomy for cystoid macular oedema with attached posterior hyaloid membrane in patients with diabetes. *Br J Ophthalmol* 1999; **83**: 12–14.

Klein R, Klein BEK, Moss SE, Davis MD, DeMets DL. The Wisconsin Epidemiologic Study of Diabetic Retinopathy. IV. Diabetic macular oedema. *Ophthalmology* 1984; **91**: 1464–74.

Lewis H, Abrams GW, Blumenkranz MS, Campo R. Vitrectomy for diabetic macular traction and oedema associated with posterior hyaloidal traction. *Ophthalmology* 1992; **99**: 753–9.

Moorman CM, Hamilton AM. Clinical applications of the MicroPulse diode laser. *Eye* 1999; **13**: 145–50.

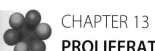

CHAPTER 13

PROLIFERATIVE DIABETIC RETINOPATHY

INTRODUCTION

The development of newly formed blood vessels either on the retina or on the optic disc, with or without fibrous tissue, signifies the presence of proliferative retinopathy. New vessels develop in response to retinal ischaemia, and the presence of neovasularization carries a high risk of significant loss of vision due to various complications:

- Vitreous haemorrhage.
- Traction upon the fovea.
- Retinal detachment.
- Neovascular glaucoma.

EPIDEMIOLOGY

The Wisconsin Epidemiological Study of Diabetic Retinopathy (WESDR) showed that the prevalence of proliferative retinopathy in type 1 diabetic patients is 0% in the first 5 years of diagnosis, increasing to 67% in those with diabetes of >35 years duration. In type 2 diabetes, the corresponding prevalence rates are 2% rising to 16% among those with diabetes for >15 years. Because type 2 diabetes is much more common, the absolute numbers of patients with proliferative eye disease is similar for the two types of diabetes. In the WESDR, approximately 43% of those examined with proliferative disease had type 1 diabetes whilst 42% had insulin-treated type 2 diabetes. The severity of proliferative disease is generally greater in type 1 diabetes, and the WESDR also showed that among patients with severe background retinopathy the 4-year incidence of proliferative retinopathy is around 40–50%.

In the Diabetic Retinopathy Study (DRS), the risk of severe visual loss (worse than 5/200) in eyes with proliferative disease was 16% over 2 years. The risk was highest in patients with new vessels on the optic disc and those with vitreous or preretinal haemorrhages. The appearance of new vessels on the retina did not further increase the risk of severe visual loss in eyes with established new vessels on the disc.

DEFINITIONS

Pathological newly formed blood vessels in the eye can be classified into three groups:

- New vessels on the retina, commonly called new vessels elsewhere (NVE), usually defined as being greater than one disc diameter from the optic disc (**Fig. 13.1**).

- New vessels on the optic disc (NVD), i.e. on the disc or within one disc diameter from the optic disc (**Fig. 13.2**).
- New vessels on the iris (**Fig. 13.3**).

DIAGNOSIS AND NATURAL HISTORY

The diagnosis of proliferative disease is made clinically after a thorough examination of the retina with mydriasis, ideally using slit-lamp biomicroscopy with a non-contact 78 or 90 dioptre lens. A three-mirror lens should be used if neovascularization of the extreme retinal periphery is suspected. The normal sequence of examination would be to firstly examine the posterior pole where neovascularization is common, arising from the optic disc or the larger vessels in the posterior pole, followed by a sequential examination of each quadrant of the retina, extending out to the periphery.

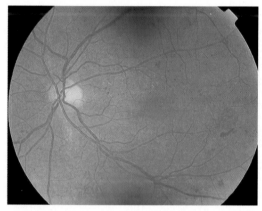

Fig. 13.1 New vessels elsewhere (NVE).

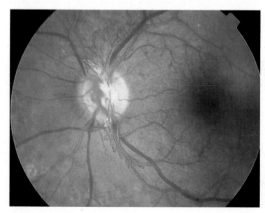

Fig. 13.2 New vessels on the optic disc (NVD).

New vessels are most frequently found within about 45 degrees of the optic disc, and NVD is present in approximately 70% of cases of proliferative disease, often in combination with NVE. Disc new vessels usually appear as fine vessels across the optic disc cup. New vessels are distinguished from normal vessels by their growth pattern and by being in a more superficial plane. They usually appear to emanate from a localized area of a retinal vein, and the size of these vessels can vary considerably.

Retinal new vessels can sometimes be difficult to differentiate from intraretinal microvascular abnormalities (IRMA). Remember that NVE are on the retinal surface and will therefore grow over retinal structures such as other blood vessels. NVE will also leak fluorescein profusely (**Fig. 13.4**).

Most new vessels eventually acquire an envelope of fibroglial tissue, and

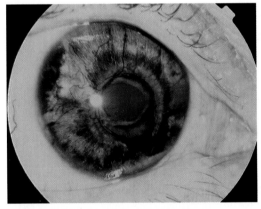

Fig. 13.3
Iris new vessels.

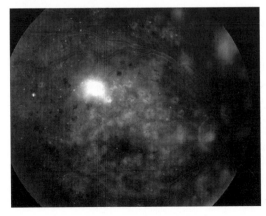

Fig. 13.4 Fluorescein angiogram revealing extensive fluorescein leakage from retinal new vessels.

in the early stages the vitreous remains adherent to both the fibrovascular tuft and the surrounding retina. Eventually, however, a localized vitreous detachment is induced around the area of fibrovascular adhesion, with the fibrovascular tissue still attached to the vitreous (the vitreous detachment is therefore incomplete). Contraction of the posterior vitreous can lead to a vitreous haemorrhage, which can be subhyaloid (preretinal, i.e. between the retina and the posterior vitreous surface), or into the body of the vitreous. The process of vitreous detachment usually occurs gradually, over months or even years, during which time multiple vitreous haemorrhages can occur.

Evidence of traction may be visible in the form of retinal tractional lines or striae, or a localized area of retinal detachment. Occasionally, a rhegmatogenous retinal detachment develops if the tractional forces produce a tear in the retina.

In the presence of a vitreous haemorrhage, fundus examination may be difficult. Consideration should be given to whether there is another cause for the vitreous haemorrhage, e.g. a retinal tear, or if there is a retinal detachment. An ultrasound examination may be helpful. Blood in the preretinal space retains its red colour but blood within the vitreous eventually takes on a yellowish-grey appearance (ochre membrane). The possibility of haemolytic or ghost-cell glaucoma needs to be considered, especially after a vitreous haemorrhage has been present for a while.

PATHOGENESIS

Retinal hypoxia due to capillary and arteriolar closure is the primary pathophysiological stimulus inducing new vessel formation. Hypoxia induces the local production of diffusible growth factors, e.g. vascular permeability factor (VPF), which initiate formation of new endothelial cells from existing blood vessels.

TREATMENT

The principal form of treatment for proliferative retinopathy remains that of panretinal laser photocoagulation or ablation. It is still unclear how panretinal laser treatment works but various hypotheses include:

- Ablation of ischaemic inner retinal tissue. Since most of the laser energy is absorbed by the retinal pigment epithelium, a heavy burn is required to destroy the inner retina from the choroid.
- Ablation of oxygen-consuming photoreceptors which lie adjacent to the retinal pigment epithelium, allowing more oxygen to diffuse further into the ischaemic inner retina.

- Destruction of the retinal pigment epithelium may release some sort of new vessel inhibiting factor.

Panretinal laser treatment is indicated for NVD and vitreous haemorrhage (**Fig. 13.5**). It should also be considered for patients with isolated NVE and those with severe preproliferative features.

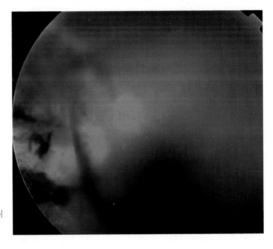

Fig. 13.5 Diffuse intragel vitreous haemorrhage.

LASER TREATMENT TECHNIQUES

The argon laser is the most widely used, but panretinal laser treatment can be applied with a krypton laser, gas laser, diode laser or the double-frequency YAG laser. For slit-lamp delivery, use a wide-angle contact lens such as the Volk Quadraspheric lens. The spot size setting is usually 200–500 µm, spaced 0.5–1.5 burn-widths apart, with a pulse duration of 0.1 seconds. The power should be set to deliver a medium intensity burn (creamy-white effect), e.g. an initial power setting for the argon laser of 200 mW for slit-lamp delivery or approximately 300 mW for delivery through the indirect ophthalmoscope. The number of laser shots may vary from 1200 to several thousand, according to severity of disease and response, and two or three treatment sessions are undertaken at weekly intervals.

It is useful at the start of treatment to delineate the macula by a line of laser burns linking the superior and inferior temporal vascular arcades. Treatment should then begin 2–3 disc diameters from the centre of the macula. It is advisable to treat the inferior retina in the first session because any subsequent vitreous haemorrhage may obscure its view. Direct laser treatment of new vessels is rarely indicated.

COMPLICATIONS OF LASER TREATMENT

- Macular oedema, which is usually transient.
- Constriction of the visual field with implications for night vision and driving.
- Retinal haemorrhage.
- Rupture of Bruch's membrane and development of a choroidal neovascular membrane.
- Suprachoroidal effusion.
- Uveitis.
- Fibrous tissue contraction precipitating a tractional retinal detachment.

Risk of these complications is minimized by using lower energy levels and applying the treatment over several sessions.

INDICATIONS FOR VITRECTOMY

Pars plana vitrectomy techniques have improved over recent years and the indications for a vitrectomy in the context of proliferative diabetic retinopathy have widened but the main ones remain: (1) persistent severe vitreous haemorrhage; and (2) tractional macular retinal detachment. The timing of a vitrectomy depends on a variety of factors, but the Diabetic Retinopathy Vitrectomy Study reported that in type 1 diabetic patients early intervention (within 6 months of a dense vitreous haemorrhage) produced better visual results compared with deferring surgery for a year. In patients with type 2 diabetes, however, deferment did not alter outcome. Other factors which may influence the timing of vitrectomy include:

- Severity of haemorrhage and prior state of the retina (the more severe the retinopathy status, the sooner surgery should be considered).
- Extent of panretinal photocoagulation before haemorrhage.
- Visual potential.
- Presence of tractional macular detachment.
- Extensive neovascularization, refractory to the effects of laser.

Additional indications for vitrectomy

- Traction on the optic disc or peripapillary retina.
- Macular traction or distortion, if macular function is otherwise good.
- Significant premacular haemorrhage, which if left untreated may produce significant fibrosis of the overlying posterior hyaloid with subsequent tractional sequelae.
- Significant fibrous proliferation anterior to the macula, reducing vision.

Complications of vitrectomy

- Retinal detachment.
- Cataract.
- Endophthalmitis.
- Elevated intraocular pressure; usually transient.
- Corneal epithelial defects.
- Persistent vitreous haemorrhage.
- Recurrent vitreous haemorrhage. This may result from residual neovascularization (or subsequent neovascularization) at the vitreous base, or from fibrovascular ingrowth through sclerotomy sites.

Visual improvement following vitrectomy has been reported in 59–83% of patients, with greater than 80% retaining a clear vitreous cavity. However, the complications following vitrectomy can be considerable and rates of no light perception have been reported at over 20%.

CURRENT ISSUES

- Laser photocoagulation remains the mainstay of treatment for proliferative diabetic retinopathy.
- Since the primary pathogenic mechanism of proliferative retinopathy is ischaemia-induced formation of growth factors, treatments that block angiogenic pathways, e.g. VPF release and action, are likely to provide effective prevention.
- Pharmacological vitreolysis may be a possible future technique for separating the vitreous from the retina.
- The indications for vitrectomy are expanding as surgical techniques improve.

FURTHER READING

Early Treatment Diabetic Retinopathy Study Research Group. Early photocoagulation for diabetic retinopathy. ETDRS report number 9. *Ophthalmology* 1991; **98**: 766–85.

Flynn HW Jr, Chew EY, Simons BD, Barton FB, Remaley NA, Ferris FL 3rd. Pars plana vitrectomy in the Early Treatment Diabetic Retinopathy Study. ETDRS report number 17. The Early Treatment Diabetic Retinopathy Study Research Group. *Ophthalmology* 1992; **99**: 1351–7.

The Diabetic Retinopathy Vitrectomy Study Research Group. Early vitrectomy for severe vitreous haemorrhage in diabetic retinopathy. *Arch Ophthalmol* 1990; **108**: 958–64.

The Diabetic Retinopathy Research Study Group. Four risk factors for severe visual loss in diabetic retinopathy: the third report from the Diabetic Retinopathy Study. *Arch Ophthalmol* 1979; **97**: 654–5.

The Early Treatment Diabetic Retinopathy Study Research Group. Techniques for scatter and local photocoagulation treatment of diabetic retinopathy: Early Treatment Diabetic Retinopathy Study Report no. 3. *Int Ophthalmol Clin* 1987; **27**: 254–64.

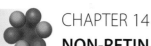

NON-RETINAL DIABETIC OCULAR COMPLICATIONS

INTRODUCTION

Whilst retinopathy is the principal ocular complication of diabetes, other associated ocular pathologies can also give rise to significant visual deficit. The following conditions have been linked with diabetes:
- Cataract formation;
- Glaucoma;
- Retinal vascular occlusion;
- Uveitis; and
- Ocular nerve palsies.

CATARACT

It is not always easy to demonstrate the exact cause of a cataract because it is a common problem, particularly in people of more advanced age. However, it is unusual for a young, otherwise healthy lens to develop a cataract and therefore a cataract in a young diabetic patient is very likely to be secondary to the presence of chronic hyperglycaemia. There is evidence of an inverse association between glycaemic control and lens clarity and, like retinopathy, rapid improvement in glycaemic control may also adversely affect the lens.

The lens opacities which occur in diabetes frequently take the form of a cortical cataract, with white dots or specks developing predominantly in the anterior and posterior subcapsular region. This form of cataract is similar to the sugar cataracts in experimental diabetic animals and is more likely to be seen in poorly controlled type 1 diabetic patients. Sugar cataracts can develop fairly rapidly, and improved control retards their progression. It is also recognized that a nuclear-sclerotic type of cataract, which is usually age related, can develop at an earlier age in patients with diabetes.

The polyol pathway has been implicated in cataract formation. Excessive amounts of intralenticular glucose becomes converted to sorbitol. Lens cell membranes and the capsule of the lens are relatively impermeable to sorbitol, raising the intralenticular osmotic pressure and affecting various intracellular metabolic pathways. This leads to an increased intake of water which causes lens cells to swell, disrupting their function and causing rupture and loss of lens clarity.

Glycation of lens proteins is another pathological mechanism that leads to cross-linking and, since the orientation of proteins is crucial to lens clarity, cataract formation. Accumulation of glycation end-products also accentuates the oxidative damage to lens proteins, especially with the lens exposed to light. A nuclear sclerotic cataract is more likely to develop following a pars plana vitrectomy for the complications of proliferative retinopathy.

The majority of patients undergoing cataract surgery will have a good visual outcome. However, the complication rate is higher in diabetic compared with non-diabetic patients. The complications of cataract extraction in patients with diabetes include:

- Increased risk of cystoid macular oedema, which is more likely to be persistent; it is therefore important to apply macular laser treatment, if possible, before contemplating cataract surgery.
- Increased risk of postoperative uveitis, especially in the presence of active proliferative retinopathy. It is therefore desirable to treat proliferative disease with panretinal laser treatment before undertaking cataract surgery, but this may not be possible because of a dense cataract, in which case laser treatment should be undertaken in the operating room with the indirect laser after cataract removal. There is some evidence that use of heparin surface-modified intraocular lenses reduces the degree of postoperative uveitis and lens surface deposition of giant cells.
- Increased incidence of iris neovascularization.
- A larger than usual anterior capsular opening should be created since the capsulotomy is more likely to contract postoperatively in patients with retinopathy.
- Increased risk of endophthalmitis.

Cataract surgery may be more difficult to perform in patients with diabetes because pupillary dilatation may be limited, there may be posterior synechiae present and the presence of iris neovascularization increases the risk of a haemorrhage peri-operatively.

GLAUCOMA

There is conflicting evidence as to whether the incidence of chronic open angle glaucoma is more common in diabetic patients. On balance, there is probably a slightly increased risk. This is in addition to the higher risk of angle-closure glaucoma in neovascular glaucoma, whereby neovascularization develops in the anterior chamber angle leading to its occlusion.

Neovascular glaucoma is a difficult condition to manage. Panretinal laser treatment should be applied if iris neovascularization is present in order to prevent neovascular glaucoma. The relatively recent introduction of laser cycloablation has added to the armementarium of treatment options.

Following a trabeculectomy, diabetic patients have an increased incidence of late-onset endophthalmitis.

RETINAL VASCULAR ABNORMALITIES

Several types of vascular abnormality are more common in patients with diabetes. These include:

- Central retinal vein occlusion (CRVO) (**Fig. 14.1**);
- Branch retinal vein occlusion (BRVO) (**Fig. 14.2**); and
- Ocular ischaemic syndrome.

These conditions can be mistaken for diabetic retinopathy, but are distinguished by the characteristic distribution of various vascular lesions, principally haemorrhages, exudates and cotton wool spots and varying degrees of retinal oedema.

In the venous occlusive diseases, the retinal veins are usually more tortuous, either generally (CRVO) or segmentally (BRVO). In CRVO, there may be varying degrees of swelling of the optic disc. It is usually possible to deter-

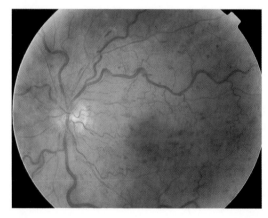

Fig. 14.1 Central retinal vein occlusion (CRVO).

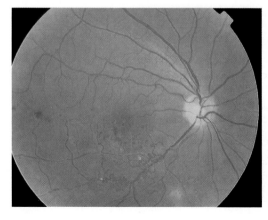

Fig. 14.2 Branch retinal vein occlusion (BRVD).

mine the presence of a collateral circulation either at the optic disc (CRVO) or at the boundaries of the area affected by a BRVO. These can sometimes be mistaken for IRMA, or neovascularization, but can usually be differentiated from each other with a fluorescein angiogram (**Fig. 14.3**).

The ocular ischaemic syndrome usually results from occlusive carotid disease and produces a combination of retinal signs which may be difficult to differentiate from diabetic retinopathy, although there may be a preponderance of cotton wool spots and vision may deteriorate rapidly in a way that is disproportionate to the degree of retinopathy. Fluorescein angiography shows that the arm-to-retina time (i.e. the time taken from injection of fluorescein to its first appearance in the retinal vessels) is significantly reduced. Carotid Doppler examination will be helpful in diagnosing abnormal flow in the carotid arteries.

UVEITIS

Uveitis in a diabetic patient may be due to ischaemia of the anterior segment, especially in the presence of iris neovascularization. A breakdown in the blood–aqueous barrier reflects increasing severity of retinopathy, giving rise to varying degrees of anterior chamber flare.

EXTERNAL OCULAR MUSCLE PALSIES

There is an increased incidence of ischaemia-related nerve palsies affecting the function of the external ocular muscles. The most commonly affected nerve is the 6th cranial nerve (abducens) giving rise to a failure of abduction and therefore producing horizontal diplopia. The 3rd and 4th cranial nerves are less frequently affected. In the majority of cases, the function of the nerve recovers fully.

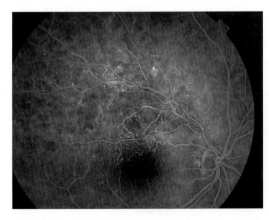

Fig. 14.3 Fluorescein angiogram in branch retinal vein occlusion demonstrating considerable collateral vessel development.

CURRENT ISSUES

- Cataract development is the commonest ocular complication in diabetes after retinopathy.
- Cataract surgery in diabetic patients with retinopathy has a higher incidence of postoperative complications, including cystoid macular oedema, uveitis and endophthalmitis. The use of heparin surface-modified intraocular lenses may lessen the severity of postoperative uveitis and the degree of giant cell deposits on the surface of the lens.
- Panretinal laser treatment in patients with active proliferative retinopathy performed before cataract surgery, or at the time or surgery using the indirect ophthalmoscope, may reduce the risk of postoperative complications.

FURTHER READING

Chew EY, Benson WE, Remaley NA *et al*. Results after lens extraction in patients with diabetic retinopathy: early treatment diabetic retinopathy study report number 25. Arch *Ophthalmol* 1999; **117**: 1600–6.

Dowler JG, Sehmi KS, Hykin PG, Hamilton AM. The natural history of macular oedema after cataract surgery in diabetes. *Ophthalmology* 1999; **106**: 663–8.

Ellis JD, Evans JM, Ruta DA *et al*. DARTS/MEMO collaboration. Diabetes Audit and Research in Tayside Study. Medicines Monitoring Unit. Glaucoma incidence in an unselected cohort of diabetic patients: is diabetes mellitus a risk factor for glaucoma? *Br J Ophthalmol* 2000; **84**: 1218–24.

Trocme SD, Li H. Effect of heparin-surface-modified intraocular lenses on postoperative inflammation after phacoemulsification: a randomized trial in a United States patient population. Heparin-Surface-Modified Lens Study Group. *Ophthalmology* 2000; **107**: 1031–7.

West JA, Dowler JG, Hamilton AM, Boyd SR, Hykin PG. Panretinal photocoagulation during cataract extraction in eyes with active proliferative diabetic eye disease. *Eye* 1999; **13**: 170–3.

QUESTIONS

1 What does this picture show?

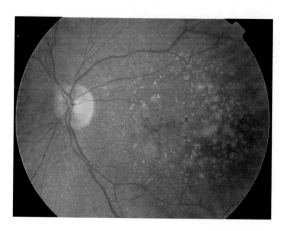

2 What is the diagnosis?

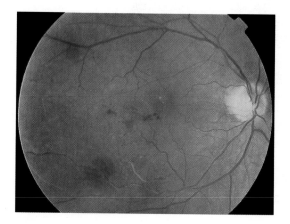

3 What is the predominant feature and what is the diagnosis?

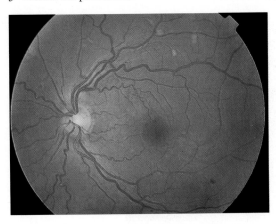

4 How should this patient be managed?

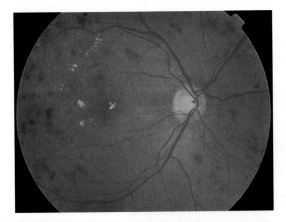

5 What is the diagnosis?

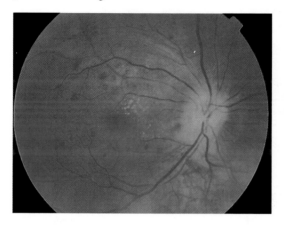

6 What does this demonstrate?

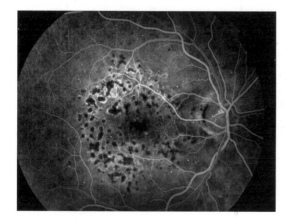

7 How should this patient be managed?

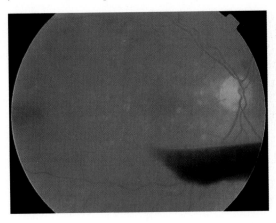

8 What is the abnormality demonstrated here?

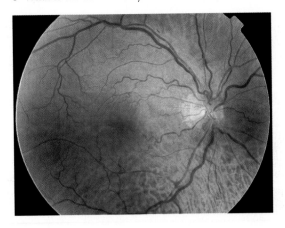

9 What is the diagnosis?

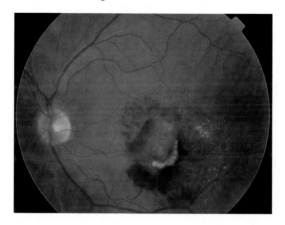

10 What is the diagnosis?

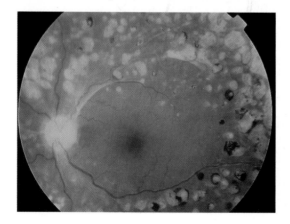

ANSWERS

Answer to Question 1
A combination of soft and hard macular drusen. Drusen generally appear softer in outline and do not have associated microaneurysms. Drusen may be considered as accumulated 'photoreceptor cell debris' and is seen with increasing frequency in the ageing eye. This patient has a few hard drusen which may be mistaken for exudates because of their harder outlines and reflective nature (this is unusual). There are also patches of pigmentation associated with age related maculopathy which may be mistaken for laser scars.

Answer to Question 2
This shows a resolving inferior branch retinal vein occlusion. Note the collateral circulation at the site of occlusion (infero-temporal) where the occluded vein is crossed over by an artery. There are also collateral vessels temporal to the macula. There are a few remaining haemorrhages and exudates at the macula. The distal portion of the occluded vessels demonstrates perivascular sheathing which is a common sequelae of retinal vein occlusion. Also note the lack of pathology in other parts of the retina with the changes confined to the quadrant supplied by the occluded vein.

Answer to Question 3
Cotton wool spots. Note also the presence of sclerotic retinal arteries with their reflective 'silver-wire' appearance and the few haemorrhages. This patient has diabetes but is also significantly hypertensive and the changes mainly reflect the effect of uncontrolled hypertension.

Answer to Question 4
There are a large number of exudates at the fovea and the multiple large deep retinal haemorrhages suggest the presence of significant degree of ischaemia. Also of significant importance is the presence of the fine vessel twigs on the superior half of the optic disc which may signify early new vessels on the optic disc (NVD). The foveal exudates are likely to indicate exudative maculopathy and this patient will probably need macular laser treatment. The disc vessels need very close supervision for signs of progression or alternatively a fluorescein angiogram could be performed to examine for signs of leakage which will confirm that they are NVD.

Answer to Question 5
This is the usual appearance of a myopic eye whereby the choroidal vasculature is usually visible (and may be mistaken for retinal neovascularization); in this

patient this is especially obvious infero-nasal to the optic disc. However, interestingly, on closer inspection, in this patient there is actually retinal neovascularization overlying this area. This picture is included here largely to demonstrate the difference between new vessels elsewhere (NVE) and normal choroidal vasculature (which is not usually visible because of shielding by the retinal pigment epithelium).

Answer to Question 6
Fluorescein angiogram of the macula highlighting laser scars applied in the form of a 'grid'; the small white spots are microaneurysms.

Answer to Question 7
This demonstrates a pre-retinal haemorrhage, i.e. blood trapped between the retina and the vitreous which is partly detached; the blood has settled to the bottom of the space created by the detached vitreous giving rise to a 'boat-shaped' haemorrhage with a fluid level. This patient may or may not be symptomatic; most are aware of a scotoma. If the haemorrhage overlies the fovea, central vision will obviously be affected. There are some new vessels located above the optic disc. This patient needs an urgent panretinal laser treatment.

Answer to Question 8
There is a collateral vessel at the optic disc which has probably resulted from a previous central retinal vein occlusion. It is not obvious from the picture but the patient also has central cystoid macular oedema.

Answer to Question 9
This patient has the exudative form of age-related macular degeneration whereby a subretinal neovascular membrane has bled giving rise to retinal and subretinal haemorrhage as well as oedema with surrounding exudates. Note the severity of the lesions and the fact that they are confined to the centre of the macula with no lesions elsewhere.

Answer to Question 10
This patient has previously had panretinal laser treatment and demonstrates regressed new vessels with remaining fibrovascular tissue. As the situation is stable, no further treatment is indicated.

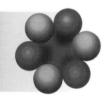

PATHOGENESIS OF GLYCAEMIC VASCULAR DYSFUNCTION

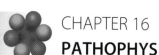

PATHOPHYSIOLOGICAL MECHANISMS

INTRODUCTION

A variety of metabolic, haemodynamic and rheological mechanisms contribute to the development and progression of micro- and macrovascular complications in patients with diabetes, but sustained exposure of vascular tissues to hyperglycaemia plays a major role in the pathogenesis of diabetic angiopathy. There is a particularly strong relationship between serum glucose levels and microvascular disease, but macrovascular events are also related to glycaemic exposure (**Fig. 16.1**). There is some debate about which marker of glycaemic control has the strongest clinical relationship with vascular disease. While fasting glucose levels and $HbA1_C$ relate closely to the incidence of diabetic retinopathy, recent evidence suggests that postprandial hyperglycaemia may be of greater prognostic value in regard to macrovascular events.

Vascular tissues exposed to high circulating levels of glucose develop a number of clinical and biochemical abnormalities, including structural and functional alterations to endothelial cells, vascular smooth muscle cells, glomeruli and mesangial cells, and cardiomyocytes. Recent studies have provided clearer insights into the underlying biochemistry and the mechanisms by which hyperglycaemia causes vascular disease. Four principal pathways are involved (**Table 16.1**).

ADVANCED GLYCOSYLATION END-PRODUCTS

A major glucose-dependent pathway of cardiovascular damage is the process of advanced glycation. This pathway involves a spontaneous, non-enzymatic reaction between glucose and NH_2-groups on tissue proteins, lipids and nucleic acids, particularly the long-lived structural proteins such as collagen, leading to the formation of advanced glycation (glycosylation) end-products (AGEs). This process involves a series of biochemical reactions (known classically as the Maillard reaction), initially resulting in the formation of Amadori (early glycation) products, the most well known example being $HbA1_C$, followed by a series of reactions generating a range of intermediates, e.g. 3-deoxyglucosone, and ultimately forming a variety of AGEs (**Fig. 16.2**).

Advanced glycation occurs over a period of weeks, and the early steps in the Maillard reaction are glucose concentration-dependent. The formation of AGEs is catalysed by transitional metals and is inhibited by antioxidant compounds such as ascorbic acid (vitamin C). If oxidation accompanies glycation, the resultant products are also known as glycoxidation products. The AGEs pentosidine and N^ε-[carboxymethyl]-lysine (CML) are examples of glycoxidation products (**Fig. 16.3**).

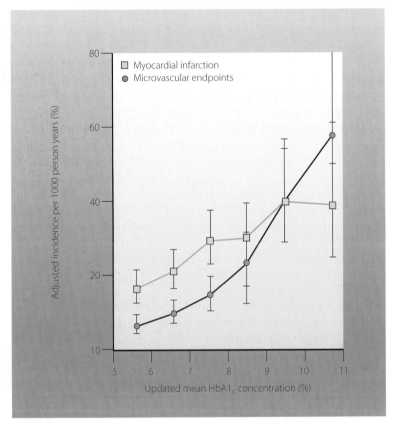

Fig. 16.1 Data from the UK Prospective Diabetes Study (UKPDS 35) showing the relationship between mean updated HbA1$_c$ concentration and the adjusted incidence (per 1000 person years) of acute myocardial infarction and microvascular endpoints. Adapted from *BMJ* 2000; **321**: 405–12.

Major pathways that have been implicated in the pathogenesis of hyperglycaemia-induced vascular injury

- Non-enzymatic glycation formation of advanced glycosylation end products (AGEs)
- Polyol pathway: aldose reductase-mediated changes in sorbitol and myoinositol
- Protein kinase C (PKC) activation: formation of diaclyglycerol and PKC activation
- Redox potential alterations: changes in free radicals and oxidation state

Table 16.1 Major pathways that have been implicated in the pathogenesis of hyperglycaemia-induced vascular injury.

The formation of reactive intermediate products during Amadori rearrangement is a crucial step in the Maillard reaction. These compounds are known as α-dicarbonyls or oxoaldehydes and include such products as 3-deoxyglucosone (3-DG) and methylglyoxal (MGO). 3-DG is formed by non-oxidative rearrangement and hydrolysis of Amadori adducts and from fructose-3-phosphate, which is a product of the polyol pathway (**Fig. 16.2**). MGO is also formed from non-oxidative mechanisms in anaerobic glycolysis and from oxidative decomposition of polyunsaturated fatty acids.

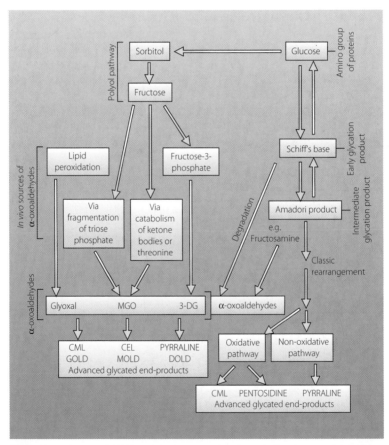

Fig. 16.2 Pathways of AGE formation incorporating the polyol pathway and AGE formation via α-oxoaldehydes. AGEs are biochemically heterogeneous but associated with a number of structural and functional abnormalities particularly involving cross-linking of long-lived structural tissue proteins, e.g. collagen. *Diabetologia* 2001; **44**: 129–146.

Carbonyl stress

MGO, 3-DG and glyoxal (collectively the α-oxoaldehydes) are formed from various steps in the glycation process via degradation of glucose or Schiff's bases in early glycation, or from Amadori products such as fructosamine in the intermediate stages of glycation (**Fig. 16.3**). Thus, α-oxoaldehydes appear to be important biochemical mediators through which glucose goes on to form AGEs by the classical Maillard reaction, the polyol pathway, as

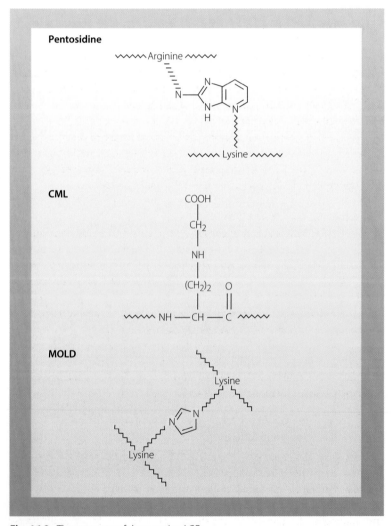

Fig. 16.3. The structure of three major AGEs.

well as from *in vivo* factors such as the catabolism of ketone bodies and threonine.

The accumulation of reactive dicarbonyl precursors is known as carbonyl stress, i.e. the accumulation of α-oxoaldehyde intermediates which may progress to form oxidative AGEs such as CML and pentosidine or non-oxidative AGEs derived from 3-DG or MGO. The process of carbonyl stress has been observed in both diabetes and end-stage renal failure, and has been implicated in the accelerated vascular damage characteristic of both conditions.

Structure of AGEs

Pentosidine and CML are the best characterized AGEs, and are often referred to as glycoxidation products (**Fig. 16.3**). Antioxidants reduce the formation of these two AGEs. In addition, lipid oxidation also plays a role in CML formation, and therefore CML appears to be a general biomarker of oxidative stress resulting from both carbohydrate and lipid oxidation reactions.

Glycation of haemoglobin forms $HbA1_C$, which has been described as an Amadori product but $HbA1_C$ is not an AGE. $HbA1_C$ is an indicator of glycaemic control for the preceding 6–12 weeks, whereas advanced glycation reflects a process that can occur over a much longer time period.

AGE and cross-link formation

Although AGEs have a variety of chemical structures, a common consequence of AGE formation is covalent cross-linking (**Table 16.2**). Structural tissue proteins, e.g. collagen, are particularly affected by the cross-link process, which mainly involves lysine residues. AGE-induced cross-link formation leads to increased stiffness of the tissue protein matrix, in part due to increased matrix protein production accompanied by decreased matrix degradation. This process has a major effect on tissue remodelling (**Table 16.2**).

Increased AGE-mediated cross-link formation occurs with advancing age and is markedly accelerated in diabetes. The physiological consequences of cross-link formation include sclerosis of renal glomeruli, thickening of the capillary basement membrane and atherosclerosis progression.

AGE receptors

Several AGE receptors have been identified, including macrophage scavenger receptor types 1 and 2, receptor for AGE (RAGE), oligosaccaharyl transferase-48 (AGE-R1), 80K-H phosphoprotein (AGE-R2) and galectin-3 (AGE-R3). These receptors are expressed on a wide range of cells including vascular smooth muscle cells, monocytes, macrophages, endothelial cells, podocytes and microglia. In particular, expression of some of these receptors is

Harmful effects of AGEs

Possible roles of AGEs and age receptors in complications of diabetes

Diabetes atherosclerosis
Vascular tissue AGE accumulation → protein cross-linking → oxidative damage
↑ Vascular matrix → thickening and narrowing of lumen
↑Endothelial cell permeability and procoagulant activity → thrombosis

Mononuclear cell chemotaxis/activation → cytokine and growth factor release:
T-cell stimulation → interferon-γ production
↑ Macrophage uptake of AGE–LDL → atheroma

Diabetic kidney disease
↑ Mesangial matrix secretion
↑ Basement membrane deposition
↑ Vascular permeability
↑ Growth factor secretion

Glomerular hypertrophy → glomerulosclerosis

Table 16.2 Harmful effects of AGEs.

increased in diabetes, e.g. AGE-R. Similarly, RAGE expression is increased in the blood vessels and kidneys of diabetic patients.

The best characterized AGE receptor is RAGE, which is a multiligand member of the immunoglobulin superfamily. Experimental studies have shown that AGE binding to the RAGE receptor on macrophages leads to oxidative stress and activation of the transcription factor NF-κB. In addition, animal studies using a soluble RAGE which blocks the RAGE receptor have shown suppression of vascular lesion formation as well as improved vascular permeability and dysfunction.

Aminoguanidine

Studies involving inhibition of AGE formation using the hydrizine derivative, aminoguanidine, have provided more direct evidence supporting the role of AGEs in diabetic vascular injury. Aminoguanidine treatment has been shown to decrease AGE formation in rat tissues, including the aorta, kidney and retina. Aminoguanidine does not inhibit the formation of early glycated products but acts at a site beyond this step (one that is not yet clearly defined), leading to reduced AGE formation.

Experimental studies have shown that aminoguanidine treatment of diabetic rats reduces microaneurysm formation and pericyte loss. In addition, beneficial effects on peripheral nerve function and structure have also been reported.

Under normal conditions, advanced glycated haemoglobin (Hb-AGE) accounts for 0.42% of circulating haemoglobin, but this increases to 0.75% in diabetic subjects. In an early clinical trial, aminoguanadine 1200 mg/day reduced levels of Hb-AGE by 28% after 1 month in subjects with diabetes for an average duration of 20 years. A related compound, pimagedine, has also been shown in clinical studies to retard the progression of diabetic nephropathy in optimally treated type 1 diabetic subjects. The side-effect profile of aminoguanidine makes it unsuitable for widespread clinical use. Early studies showed changes in the blood film resembling pernicious anaemia, but of greater concern is the development of antinuclear antibodies and clinical features of vasculitus and glomerulonephritis.

New, more potent inhibitors of advanced glycation have been developed recently, including ALT-462 and ALT-486, which are approximately five- and 20-fold more potent than aminoguanidine *in vitro*. In addition, the cross-link breaker, PTB, is a thiazolium compound which cleaves di-ketone bridges between adjacent carbonyl groups. Daily intraperitoneal injections of PTB in STZ-diabetic rats have been shown to ameliorate AGE-induced cross-links. Pyridoxamine (also known as pyridorin) is another pharmacological inhibitor of the conversion of Amadori intermediates to AGEs. Similarly, the compound OPB-9195 reduces AGE accumulation in glomeruli of experimental diabetic rats, in part through suppression of TGF-β and VEGF expression.

THE POLYOL PATHWAY

In this metabolic pathway, glucose is reduced to sorbitol by the enzyme aldose reductase (**Fig. 16.4**). Under physiological conditions of normoglycaemia, the polyol pathway plays a very minor role in glucose disposal, but in diabetic states vascular cells undergoing insulin-dependent glucose uptake produce increased amounts of sorbitol which is slowly metabolized to fructose. The accumulation of sorbitol inside vascular cells results in osmotic stress, decreased myoinositol content, abnormal phosphoinositide metabolism, and decreased Na^+/K^+-ATPase activity.

The polyol pathway and formation of sorbitol have been implicated in diabetic complications, including retinopathy, neuropathy, cataracts, nephropathy and corneal disease. In experimental animals, inhibition of aldose reductase leads to reduced neuropathy, and prevention of myoinositol depletion and reduced ATPase activity in the kidney. Other experimental studies have shown that aldose reductase inhibition produces significant reductions in proteinuria and other markers of diabetic nephropathy in animal models.

Unfortunately, clinical studies using aldose reductase inhibitors over the past 20 years have been disappointing and this therapeutic approach has been largely abandoned as an option for preventing diabetic vascular dysfunction.

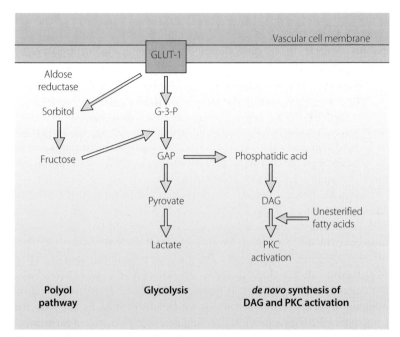

Fig. 16.4. Glucose enters vascular cells via the GLUT-1 transporter, and most glucose undergoes glycolysis with a minor component (<5%) entering the polyol pathway. Under conditions of hyperglycaemia and increased glycolysis, glyceraldehyde-3-phosphate (GAP) is converted to phosphatidic acid, which in turn results in increased *de novo* synthesis of diacylglycerol (DAG). Newly synthesized DAG is rich in palmitate, which preferentially activates the PKC-β isoforms in vascular cells. Unesterified free fatty acids augment DAG-mediated PKC activation.

CURRENT ISSUES

- Defining the biochemical pathways involved in AGE formation, and the mechanisms of AGE-induced protein cross-linking, will lead to the identification of new pharmacological approaches that mimic the profile of aminoguanidine but have acceptable safety characteristics for routine clinical practice. A number of compounds are in development.
- Experimental studies have clearly suggested that oxidative stress plays an important part in the vascular damage associated with AGE formation and PKC activation, but so far clinical trials of vitamin C and vitamin E supplementation have been disappointing in terms of reducing cardiovascular events.
- Aldose reductase inhibitors have been largely disappointing in clinical trials, perhaps because only 5% of glucose transported into vascular cells, even under conditions of hyperglycaemia, passes through the polyol pathway.

FURTHER READING

Idris I, Gray S, Donnelly R. Protein kinase C activation: isozyme-specific effects on metabolism and cardiovascular complications in diabetes. *Diabetologia* 2001; **44**: 659–673.

Singh R, Barden A, Mori T, Beilin L. Advanced glycation end products: A review. *Diabetologia* 2001; **44**: 129–46.

Tsuchida K, Makita Z, Yamagishi S *et al.* Suppression of transforming growth factor β and vascular endothelial growth factor in diabetic nephropathy in rats by a novel AGE inhibitor, OPB-9195. *Diabetologia* 1999; **42**: 579–88.

PROTEIN KINASE C

INTRODUCTION

It is now recognized that activation of protein kinase C (PKC) under conditions of hyperglycaemia is one of the principal mechanisms of vascular damage in patients with diabetes. Glucose is transported into vascular cells by GLUT-1 transporters and then metabolized, mostly via glycolysis (<5% is metabolized by the aldose reductase/polyol pathway, even under conditions of hypergly-caemia). GLUT-1 expression in vascular cells is up-regulated by high extracel-lular glucose concentrations and other local factors involved in diabetic angiopathy, e.g. hypoxia. The increase in glycolysis results in increased *de novo* synthesis of diacylglycerol (DAG), which is the main endogenous activator of a ubiquitous intracellular enzyme known as PKC. Several studies have shown both in animals and humans with diabetes that there is a widespread increase in DAG levels and PKC activity in different types of vascular cell (**Table 17.1**).

PKC: A MULTIFUNCTIONAL FAMILY OF ISOENZYMES

It has long been recognized that adding and removing phosphate groups is one of the most important physiological mechanisms by which the activity of cellular proteins (e.g. enzymes and receptors) is regulated. For example, key

Diabetes-related activation of DAG-PKC pathway in vascular cells and tissues				
	Species	DAG Content	PKC Activity	Isoforms Activated
Cells in Culture				
Aortic Endothelial	Rat, bovine	↑	↑	β
Aortic VSM	Rat, human	↑	↑	-β
Retinal Endothelial	Bovine	↑	↑	-βII, -δ
Retinal Pericytes	Bovine	NM	↑	-βII, -δ
Renal mesangial	Rat	↑	↑	-α, βI
Renal glomerular	Rat	↑	↑	-α, βI
Tissues				
Heart	Rat, human	↑	↑	-β, -ε
Retina	Rat, canine	↑	↑	-βII, δ
Aorta	Rat, canine	↑	↑	-β
Glomeruli	Rat, mouse	↑	↑	-δ, -βI, -α
Monocytes	Human	NM	↑	-βII

↑ = increased; NM = not measured

Table 17.1 Diabetes-related activation of DAG–PKC pathway in vascular cells and tissues.

metabolic enzymes such as glycogen synthase are switched on and off by intracellular kinases (enzymes that add phosphate groups) and phosphatases (enzymes that remove phosphate groups), which are themselves regulated by other biochemical signals, e.g. hormones and growth factors.

Intracellular kinases are broadly divided into two different types: those that phoshorylate proteins at tyrosine residues (known as tyrosine kinases) and those that phoshorylate serine and threonine sites (known as serine/threonine kinases). There are two major serine/threonine kinases that are widely distributed in all tissues: cyclic-AMP- dependent protein kinase (also known as protein kinase A) and PKC.

PKC was first described over 20 years ago as a single, proteolytically activated kinase, and cancer biologists were the first to take a keen interest in this enzyme because early studies showed that tumour-promoting substances known as phorbol esters caused prolonged activation of PKC. Since then, however, it has become clear that PKC plays an important regulatory role in a variety of cellular responses, in addition to cell growth and differentiation, and that PKC is involved in gene expression, secretion of hormones and postreceptor signalling. Thus, PKC phosphorylates (and thereby regulates) a large number of intracellular substrates, including proteins such as the insulin receptor and key metabolic enzymes involved in glucose transport and utilization.

Although PKC was first described as a single enzyme, molecular and genetic studies over the last 10 years have shown that PKC is in fact a family of structurally and functionally related proteins which are derived from multiple genes (at least three) and from alternative splicing of single mRNA transcripts. Twelve isoenzymes of PKC have so far been cloned and characterized. They are classified into three groups according to their structural homologies (**Table 17.2**). Individual isoforms have different patterns of tissue distribution, substrate specificity and cofactor requirements. For example, the group A (classical) PKC isoforms (PKC-α, -β_I and -β_{II}) require the presence of both calcium and phospholipid for enzyme activation, whereas the group B (novel) PKC isoforms are calcium-independent and group C (atypical) PKC isoforms are both calcium- and phospholipid-independent (**Table 17.2**).

The brain and liver contain virtually all PKCs, but most other tissues express only certain PKC isoforms. The different patterns of tissue expression reflect a complex multifunctional role for this family of kinases, but specific functions related to individual isoenzymes are incompletely understood. Activation and translocation of PKC in vascular cells correlates with circulating glucose concentrations, as illustrated in a recent clinical study using monocytes (**Fig. 17.1**).

EFFECTS OF DIABETES ON DAG-PKC ACTIVATION IN VASCULAR TISSUES

Several studies have clearly demonstrated increased tissue levels of DAG and isoform-selective activation of PKC in a range of vascular cell types under conditions of clinical or experimental diabetes (**Table 17.1**). Increased intra-

Protein kinase C Isoforms		
Type	**Isoform**	**Distribution**
Conventional (c) Ca** and	α	Widespread
Phospholipid-dependent	β	Widespread
	γ	Brain
Novel (n) Ca** independent	δ	Widespread
	ε	Brain, hematopoietic tissue
	η	Heart, skin, lung
	θ	Hematopoietictissue, skeletal muscle, brain
	μ	Lung, epithelial cells
Atpical (a) Ca** independent	ζ	Widespread
	ν/λ	Kidney, brain, lung

Table 17.2 Protein kinase isoforms.

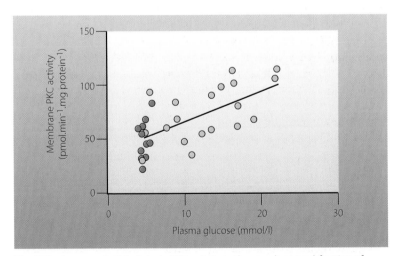

Fig. 17.1 In a recent clinical study, PKC activity in the membrane subfraction of circulating monocytes was measured in 19 patients with diabetes (●) and 14 non-diabetic control subjects (●) and showed a linear correlation with circulating plasma glucose levels ($r^2 = 0.4$, $P = 0.0001$). Adapted from *Diabetes* 1999; **48**: 1316–22.

cellular release of DAG in response to high circulating glucose concentrations is the primary step leading to activation and translocation of PKC. Various species of DAG (varying in fatty acid composition) are generated from four principal sources (**Fig. 17.2**): (1) classical receptor-mediated, phospholipase C-catalysed hydrolysis of inositol phospholipids; (2) release of DAG from phospholipase D-mediated hydrolysis of phosphatidylcholine (PC); (3) via release of free fatty acids (FFAs) from precursor lipids by the action of phospholipase A_2; and (4) *de novo* synthesis of DAG from phosphatidic acid (PA). This latter pathway is mainly responsible for hyperglycaemia-induced DAG formation in a range of cardiovascular tissues, but high glucose levels also increase the turnover of phosphatidylcholine (PC). The excess DAGs that accumulate in diabetic vascular tissues are particularly rich in the FFA palmitate which suggests that pathways 2 and 4 are the principal sources of hyperglycaemia-induced DAG formation.

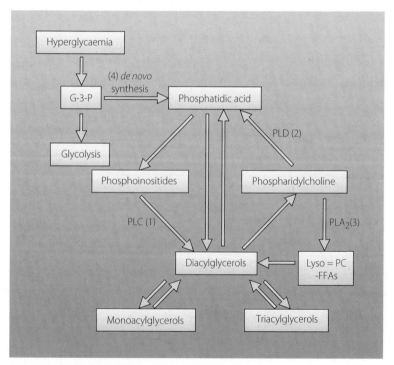

Fig. 17.2 Four principal pathways are involved in the generation of diacylglycerols in vascular tissues, but under conditions of hyperglycaemia *de novo* synthesis (4) and hydrolysis of phosphatidylcholine (2) are particularly important. See text for further details.

Experimental studies have also shown that DAG-mediated activation of PKC is augmented by specific FFAs of varying chain lengths. For example, unesterified fatty acids and their CoA esters (especially arachidonic, oleic, linoleic and linolenic acids) appear to activate PKC synergistically with DAG (**Fig. 17.3**), and it has been suggested that *cis*-unsaturated fatty acids act as 'PKC enhancer' molecules. Thus, in diabetes increased FFA levels, particularly in the postprandial state, may enhance hyperglycaemia-induced PKC activation, independently of (and in addition to fuelling) *de novo* synthesis of DAG.

There is evidence that different species of DAG preferentially activate one or more PKC isoforms in different tissues, and George King's Group at the Joslyn Diabetes Centre in Boston, USA, first made the important observation that PKC isoforms are differentially up-regulated in different tissues in

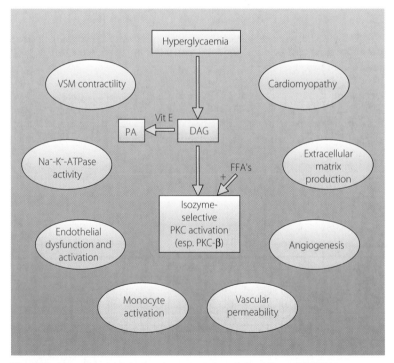

Fig. 17.3 Hyperglycaemia-induced accumulation of diacylglycerol (DAG) is ameliorated, in part, by vitamin E supplementation, which activates DAG kinase. Free fatty acids augment DAG-induced activation of specific PKC isoforms, especially PKC-β, which in turn leads to a number of important pathophysiological mechanisms involved in the structural and functional abnormalities associated with diabetic cardiovascular disease.

response to hyperglycaemia. In particular, they showed that increased activity of PKC-β is the dominant PKC response in macrovascular and renal tissues, including vascular smooth muscle and endothelial cells, as well as the retina. Furthermore, PKC-β_{II} seems to be the main PKC isoform activated in vascular tissues in response to high glucose levels, whereas in glomerular cells PKC-β_I is the predominant isoform activated by hyperglycaemia (**Fig. 17.4**).

ACTIVATION OF PKC-B

The pathophysiological consequences of PKC activation in vascular tissues will be addressed in detail in the next two chapters, but it seems clear that hyperglycaemia-induced formation of certain species of DAG leads to preferential activation of PKC-β_{II} in vascular tissues, including the retina, and preferential activation of PKC-β_I in glomerular and mesangial cells within the kidney. Activation and translocation of these isoforms from the cytosol to the plasma membrane correlates with plasma glucose levels (**Fig. 17.1**) and leads to a number of undesirable pathophysiological changes involving membrane transport, gene transcription and local vasoactive hormone secretion/responsiveness (**Fig. 17.3**).

VITAMIN E

It has been shown that the accumulation of DAG in vascular tissues in hyperglycaemic states is ameliorated, in part, by D-α-tocopherol (vitamin E), which

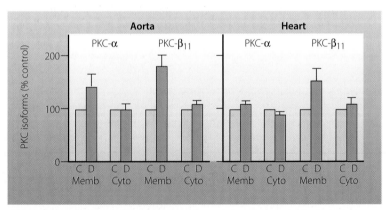

Fig. 17.4 In diabetic animal models it was shown that individual PKC isoforms are differentially up-regulated under conditions of hyperglycaemia. In particular, in the aorta and heart, PKC-β_{II} was increased to a greater extent than PKC-α in the cellular membrane fraction. Adapted from *Proc Natl Acad Sci* 1992; **89**: 11059–63.

activates DAG kinase and promotes the conversion of DAG to PA (**Fig. 17.3**). Several experimental studies have shown that glucose-induced PKC activation is attenuated by vitamin E therapy, and that the functional consequences of PKC activation in the kidney and retina are reversed. This raises the possibility that vitamin E has therapeutic benefits via reducing the DAG–PKC pathway in diabetic vascular tissues.

CURRENT ISSUES

- Hyperglycaemia-induced activation of PKC, especially PKC-β, appears to be a major pathway in the development of structural and functional abnormalities of vascular tissues in diabetes. Reducing the accumulation of DAG using vitamin E supplementation, combined with selective PKC isoenzyme inhibition, provides a logical therapeutic approach to ameliorating and reversing diabetic microangiopathy, especially in the eyes and kidneys.
- Numerous protein substrates are phosphorylated and thereby regulated in response to PKC activation, which in turn results in changes in cell growth and differentiation; contractile function; matrix production; vascular permeability; and neo-vascularization.
- Different species of DAG (varying in fatty acid composition) seem to activate different PKC isoforms in various tissues, and there is particular interest in the clinical relationships between meal-related increases in glucose and triglyceride levels, PKC activation and diabetic vascular disease.

FURTHER READING

Hug H & Sarre TF. Protein kinase C isoenzymes: divergence in signal transduction? *Biochem J* 1993; **291**: 329–43.

Inoguchi T, Battan R, Handler E *et al.* Preferential elevation of protein kinase C isoform β_{II} and diacylglycerol levels in the aorta and heart of diabetic rats. Differential reversibility to glycaemic control by islet transplantation. *Proc Natl Acad Sci USA* 1992; **89**: 11059–63.

Newton AC. Protein kinase C: structure, function and regulation; mini review. *J Biol Chem* 1995; **270**: 28495–8.

Xia P, Inoguchi T, Kern TS *et al.* Characterization of the mechanism for the chronic activation of diacylglycerol- protein kinase C pathway in diabetes and hypergalactosaemia. *Diabetes* 1994; **43**: 1122–9.

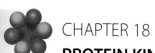

PROTEIN KINASE C ACTIVATION AND VASCULAR PERMEABILITY

INTRODUCTION

The vascular endothelium is a multifunctional barrier between the intravascular and tissue compartments; it is much more than an inert lining of blood vessels. Endothelial cells have antiadhesive and anticoagulant properties, modulate the effects of vasoconstrictor agonists, and through tight intercellular junctions control the permeability to large circulating molecules. Leakage of macromolecules through the endothelial barrier is an early feature of diabetic microvascular disease and responsible for the increase in urinary albumin excretion rate (UAE) and the typical exudative changes in diabetic retinopathy. More importantly, increased endothelial permeability—as indicated clinically by a raised UAE—confers a substantial increase in cardiovascular risk. Studies such as the WHO Multinational Study of Vascular Disease in Diabetes showed a clear relationship between proteinuria and reduced survival in both type 1 and type 2 diabetes (**Fig. 18.1**).

Thus, endothelial barrier dysfunction is an early hallmark of widespread microvascular damage, but is also indicative of increased morbidity and mor-

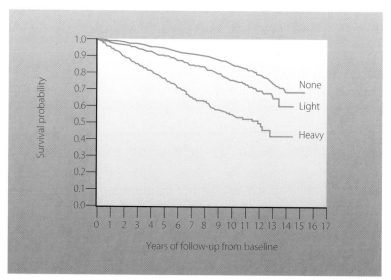

Fig. 18.1 Survival according to the degree of proteinuria (non-, slight or heavy) at baseline among patients with type 2 diabetes. Reproduced with permission from *Diabetic Medicine* 1995; **12**: 149–55.

tality from macrovascular complications. Metabolic and haemodynamic abnormalities are responsible for the increases in endothelial permeability in patients with diabetes, but high glucose levels, in particular, via activation of protein kinase C (PKC), increase vascular permeability.

MECHANISMS OF INCREASED ENDOTHELIAL PERMEABILITY

The transport of fluid and solute across the endothelial barrier is governed by filtration pressure (i.e. 'Starling forces') and the local generation of cell-derived mediators that influence endothelial barrier function. Several morphological and functional abnormalities of endothelial cells are associated with increases in vascular permeability.

Intercellular gaps

Adjacent endothelial cells form junctional complexes consisting of tight junctions and adherence junctions which are the sites of diffusional transport of solutes from the vascular to the interstitial space. The increase in *trans*-endothelial permeability in response to pro-inflammatory mediators such as histamine and thrombin can occur via contraction or retraction of cells and the resultant formation of interendothelial cell gaps. 'Rounding up' of endothelial cells is a characteristic morphological change associated with widening of the intercellular junctions and increased *trans*-endothelial albumin flux. Intracellular contractile proteins such as F-actin in the microfilaments are responsible for the shape change of endothelial cells in response to inflammatory mediators such as histamine and thrombin.

Endothelial cell contraction vs. retraction

The characteristic shape change of endothelial cells in response to inflammatory stimuli involves contraction of microfilaments within the cytoskeleton. In particular, phosphorylation of a key enzyme, myosin light chain kinase (MLCK), regulates the intracellular actin–myosin contractile mechanism. PKC plays an important role in phosphorylating MLCK and other acting-regulating proteins such as vinculin and talin which are important for maintaining cell–cell and cell–matrix contacts.

Activation of PKC by phorbol esters causes reorganization of actin and vinculin and disruption of junctional complexes in epithelial cells, consistent with the notion that PKC-dependent phosphorylation of actin-binding proteins is a critical signalling event responsible for shape change and loss of endothelial barrier function (**Fig. 18.2**). PKC also phosphorylates caldesmon and vimentin, two other cytoskeletal proteins in endothelial cells that are important for cell shape change.

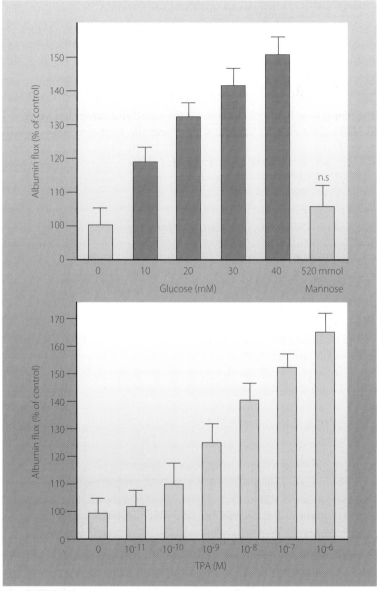

Fig. 18.2 Data showing the effects of different concentrations of glucose (upper panel) and the phorbol ester TPA (lower panel) on albumin flux across aortic endothelial monolayers. High glucose and phorbol ester-induced PKC activation are associated with dose-dependent increases in endothelial permeability. Adapted from *Circulation Research* 1997; **81**: 363–71.

HIGH-GLUCOSE-INDUCED HYPERPERMEABILITY

Several mechanisms are involved in hyperglycaemia-induced hyperpermeability:

- Increased formation of vascular permeability factor (VPF) (**Fig. 18.3**).
- Advanced glycation end-product (AGE)-mediated oxidative stress.
- Intracellular calcium release and activation of nitric oxide synthase (NOS).
- PKC activation and phosphorylation of intracellular contractile proteins, e.g. MLCK.

The biochemical mechanisms of glucose-induced hyperpermeability are not clearly understood, but activation of PKC plays an important role in each of the above pathways (Fig. 18.2). For example, PKC inhibition blocks glucose-induced over-expression of VPF (**Fig. 18.4**).

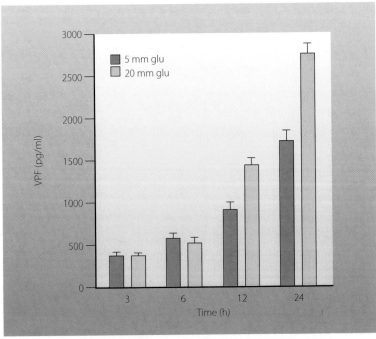

Fig. 18.3 Vascular permeability factor (VPF) plays an important role in retinal and glomerular protein leakage. Hyperglycaemia increases VPF peptide production by human vascular smooth muscle cells. VPF concentration in the culture media overlying human vascular smooth muscle (VSM) cells was determined using a specific ELISA after incubation of the cell mono-layers with control (glucose 5 mmol/l, purple bars) or high glucose medium (glucose 20 mmol/l, orange bars) for up to 24 hours Reproduced from *Diabetes* 1997; **46**: 1497–1503.

PKC ACTIVATION AND ENDOTHELIAL PERMEABILITY

Activation and translocation of PKC in endothelial cells has been associated with the hyperpermeability responses to a number of circulating factors, including thrombin, histamine and H_2O_2. In addition, non-specific PKC inhibitors such as H-7 block increases in *trans*-endothelial permeability in response to thrombin and H_2O_2. Thus, PKC activation appears to be a critical intracellular signalling event mediating the increase in endothelial permeability associated with a range of circulating factors (apart from hyperglycaemia).

An increase in intracellular calcium concentration seems to be an important trigger in endothelial cell permeability, in part via activation of calcium-dependent PKC isoforms. PKC-α and PKC-β isoforms are the predominant calcium-dependent PKC isoforms in endothelial cells, and elegant work using antisense oligonucleotides to PKC-β_1 in human microvascular endothelial cells has shown that this isoform plays a critical role in phorbol ester-induced hyperpermeability (**Fig. 18.5**). Similarly, in bovine pulmonary microvascular endothelial cells, H_2O_2 increased the *trans*-endothelial permeability to albu-

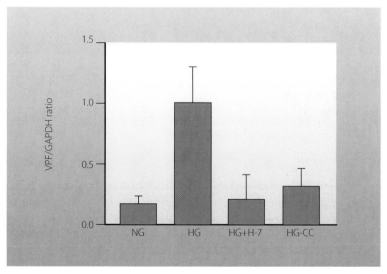

Fig. 18.4 Hyperglycaemia stimulates increased gene expression for VPF, and this pathway is PKC-dependent. These data show VPF mRNA expression (relative to a housekeeping gene, GAPDH) under conditions of normal glucose (NG), high glucose (HG) and high glucose in combination with the non-specific PKC inhibitors, H-7 and chelerythrine chloride (CC). Reproduced with permission from *Diabetes* 1997; **46**: 1497–1503.

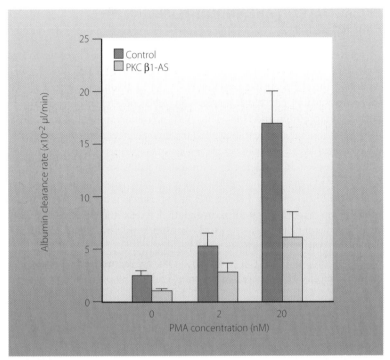

Fig. 18.5 Human microvascular endothelial cells were transfected with retroviral vectors containing the antisense oligonucleotide for PKC-β_1. Knockout of PKC-β_1 attenuated the increase in albumin permeability induced by the phorbol ester PMA (an exogenous, non-specific PKC activator), confirming that PKC-β_1 is a critical PKC isoform involved in PKC-dependent hyperpermeability responses. PKC, protein kinase C. Adapted from *J Cell Physiol* 1995; **166**: 249–55.

min in parallel with increased translocation of PKC-β to the plasma membrane, suggesting that PKC-β activation mediates the H_2O_2-induced permeability response. Thus, several experimental studies indicate that the calcium requirement for the increase in endothelial permeability may be related to a requirement for activation of calcium-dependent PKC isoforms, particularly PKC-β.

The importance of PKC in vascular permeability has been emphasized in other clinical conditions apart from diabetes, e.g. pre-eclampsia. Serum from pre-eclamptic women increased endothelial permeability *in vitro* in parallel with increased translocation of classic PKC isoforms. Furthermore, the hyperpermeability response to serum from pre-eclamptic women was attenuated using a non-specific PKC inhibitor.

CURRENT ISSUES

* A rise in intracellular calcium, combined with activation of calcium-dependent PKC isoforms, especially PKC-α and PKC-β, serves as a common biochemical signalling pathway in the hyperpermeability responses of endothelial cells to a variety of circulating factors, especially high-glucose and VPF.
* Hyperglycaemia stimulates the gene expression for VPF, a pathway that is blocked by PKC inhibitors, and VPF has been strongly implicated in the pathogenesis of exudative diabetic retinopathy.
* Restoring endothelial barrier function in patients with diabetes and microvascular complications, e.g. with blood pressure lowering therapy, seems to improve cardiovascular outcome, but novel therapeutic approaches such as PKC inhibition would augment conventional blood pressure and glucose-lowering strategies for ameliorating microangiopathy.

FURTHER READING

Bonnardel-Phu E, Wautier JL, Schmidt AM et al. Acute modulation of albumin microvascular leakage by advanced glycation end products in microcirculation of diabetic rats *in vivo. Diabetes* 1999; **48**: 2052–8.

Huang Q & Yuan Y. Interaction of PKC and NOS in signal transduction of microvascular hyperpermeability. *Am J Physiol* 1997; **273**: H2442-H2451.

Haller H, Hempel A, Homuth V et al. Endothelial-cell permeability and protein kinase C in pre-eclampsia. *Lancet* 1998; **351**: 945–9.

Hempel A et al. High glucose concentrations increase endothelial cell permeability via activation of protein kinase C-α. *Circ Res* 1997; **81**: 363–71.

Hinder F et al. Nitric oxide and endothelial permeability. *J Appl Phsiol* 1997; **83**: 1941–194.

Kuroki T et al. High glucose induces alteration of gap junction permeability and phosphorylation of connexin-43 in cultured aortic smooth muscle cells. *Diabetes* 1998; **47**: 931–6.

Lum H et al. Mechanisms of increased endothelial permeability. *Can J Physiol Pharmacol* 1996; **74**: 787–800.

Nagpala PG et al. PKC-β_1 over expression augments phorbol ester-induced increase in endothelial permeability. *J Cell Physiol* 1995; **166**: 249–55.

Siflinger-Birnboim A et al. Activation of protein kinase C pathway contributes to hydrogen peroxide-induced increase in endothelial permeability. *Laboratory Invest* 1992; **67**: 24–30.

Williams B et al. Glucose-induced protein kinase C activation regulates vascular permeability factor mRNA expression and peptide production by human vascular smooth muscle cells *in vitro. Diabetes* 1997; **46**: 1497–1503.

CHAPTER 19

HARMFUL EFFECTS OF PROTEIN KINASE C ACTIVATION IN CARDIOVASCULAR AND RENAL TISSUES

INTRODUCTION

In clinical practice, metabolic and haemodynamic abnormalities contribute to the initiation and progression of diabetic vascular complications but hyperglycaemia is particularly important in the pathogenesis of microangiopathy. Hyperglycaemia-induced *de-novo* synthesis of diacylglycerol (DAG) and isoform-selective activation of protein kinase C (PKC), especially PKC-β, plays a major role in the development of structural and functional abnormalities in vascular tissues, particularly the retina, glomerulus and vascular endothelium. Individual isoforms of PKC vary in their tissue distribution, cofactor requirements for activation, and substrates, but PKC-mediated phosphorylation of various intracellular enzymes, receptors and transcription factors adversely affects tissue function under conditions of sustained hyperglycaemia.

The mechanisms by which PKC activation in vascular tissues causes structural and functional abnormalities associated with diabetic microangiopathy are incompletely understood, but several key pathways have been identified in experimental models of diabetic retinopathy, nephropathy and endothelial dysfunction (**Fig. 19.1**).

PKC-MEDIATED CHANGES IN GENE EXPRESSION

Experimental evidence showing coactivation of PKC and mitogen-activated protein (MAP) kinases in vascular cells grown in high glucose conditions strongly suggests that these two biochemical pathways are linked. Indeed, there is now good evidence showing that activation of PKC leads to activation of MAP kinases, which in turn phosphorylate and regulate transcription factors leading to up-regulation of mRNA and protein production for a range of key intracellular proteins. In particular, PKC-mediated increases in vascular permeability factor (VPF) expression in the eye play an important role in the permeability and neo-vascularization changes seen in diabetic maculopathy and proliferative retinopathy. In addition, increased mesangial expression of transforming growth factor-β (TGFβ) leads to increases in glomerular matrix protein production, particularly fibronectin and type IV collagen. PKC activation also influences the expression of genes coding for other growth factors and metalloproteinase enzymes involved in the degradation of matrix proteins.

Thus, PKC activation, in part via MAP kinase activation, leads to up-regulation of a cluster of genes involved in the formation of structural proteins, growth factors and peptides such as VPF and TGFβ which play a pivotal role in the development of endothelial hyperpermeability, angiogenesis and matrix deposition.

ENDOTHELIAL AND VASCULAR SMOOTH MUSCLE FUNCTION

It is well established that PKC enzyme activity in endothelial and vascular smooth muscle (VSM) cells increases in relationship to the ambient glucose concentration (**Fig. 19.2**). Furthermore, glucose-stimulated PKC activation involves multiple PKC isoforms, especially the conventional PKC isoforms, e.g. PKC-β, which in turn affect vascular tone, local blood flow and the formation of platelet-derived and endothelial-derived vasodilator molecules, including nitric oxide.

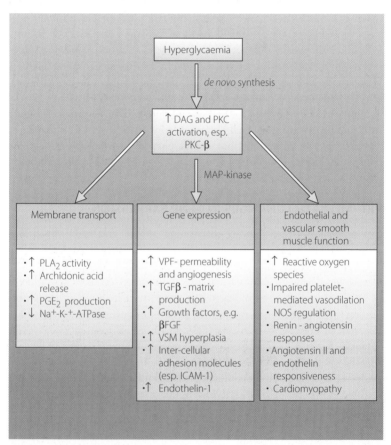

Fig. 19.1 Hyperglycaemia, via increased *de novo* synthesis of DAG and activation of several PKC isoforms, especially PKC-β, leads to various unwanted pathological effects which can be broadly grouped under three headings: increased gene expression; changes in endothelial and vascular smooth muscle (VSM) function; and altered membrane transport.

Formation of reactive oxygen species

Local formation of reactive oxygen species (ROS) by endothelial and VSM cells initiates a host of unwanted effects, and free radical generation has been implicated in various pathological changes associated with diabetic vascular disease. Formation of ROS involves activation of intracellular enzymes, e.g. NADPH oxidase and xanthine oxidase, but recent evidence has shown that high glucose levels, via activation of PKC, stimulate ROS formation by VSM and endothelial cells, a pathway that is blocked by PKC inhibitors (**Fig. 19.3**). Thus, oxidative stress, a well established feature of diabetic vascular disease, is associated with hyperglycaemia via a PKC-dependent pathway in both endothelial and smooth muscle cells. In addition, ROS-induced apoptosis of VSM cells is also PKC-dependent.

Nitric oxide synthase

The local generation of nitric oxide (NO) from the oxidation of L-arginine is catalysed by a family of nitric oxide synthases (NOS). Release of NO mediates the vasodilator responses to a number of important molecules, including acetylcholine, bradykinin and substance P, and NO-mediated vasodilation is impaired in patients with type 1 and type 2 diabetes. This is likely to reflect both reduced NO availability and reduced NO responsiveness of VSM.

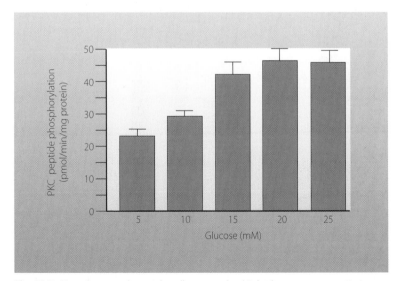

Fig. 19.2 Vascular smooth muscle cells exposed to high glucose concentrations show proportional increases in PKC enzyme activity and translocation of PKC to the plasma membrane. Data from *Diabetes* 1992; **41**: 1464–72, with permission.

Three separate genes encode the known isoforms of NOS: endothelial NOS (eNOS) and neuronal NOS (nNOS) catalyse the constitutive production of NO via a calcium-dependent pathway in blood vessels and neural tissues, respectively, while the third NOS isoform, inducible NOS (iNOS), is located in macrophages and catalyses NO formation in inflammatory cells.

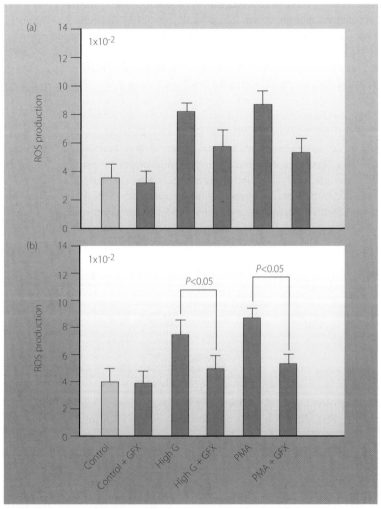

Fig. 19.3 Experimental data showing the effects of PKC inhibitors (GFX or calphostin C, CAL) on high glucose or phorbol ester (PMA) induced increases in ROS production in cultured aortic vascular smooth muscle cells (a), or endothelial cells (b). Adapted from *Diabetes* 2000; **49**: 1939–45.

There is good evidence that specific PKC isoforms regulate iNOS expression in macrophages and VSM cells. However, it would seem that different PKC isoforms can regulate iNOS in both a positive and negative manner. In addition, experimental evidence has shown that elevated glucose levels impair endothelial-dependent relaxation via PKC activation.

Impaired platelet-mediated vasodilation

Activated normal platelets produce local vasodilation via release of platelet-derived adenosine diphosphate (ADP), which in turn stimulates the release of endothelium-derived NO. NO causes VSM relaxation and inhibits platelet aggregation and excessive thrombus formation. Several studies have shown that platelets from patients with diabetes lack the ability to produce NO-dependent vasodilation. Furthermore, this defect can be reproduced experimentally by exposing normal human platelets to high glucose concentrations.

Experimental evidence would suggest that this defect is PKC-dependent. For example, platelets from patients with diabetes that were treated with a PKC inhibitor, calphostin-C, produced normal vasodilation, while untreated platelets from the same patients lacked the ability to cause vasorelaxation (**Fig. 19.4a**). Similarly, normal platelets incubated in high glucose conditions lost their ability to cause vasorelaxation, but coincubation with calphostin-C prevented glucose-mediated impairment of platelet-mediated vasodilation (**Fig. 19.4b**).

Monocyte adhesion

Binding of circulating moncytes to endothelial cells is an important early event in atheroma formation and one that is enhanced in diabetes. A recent clinical study has shown that membrane-associated PKC activity is increased in monocytes from diabetic patients and that total PKC activity, and expression of the glucose-sensitive PKC-β isoform, decreased by 40% under normoglycaemic conditions. Because increased PKC activity in monocytes enhances their adhesion to the vascular wall, increases fibrinogen binding and promotes differentiation into macrophages, augmentation of this signal transduction pathway could well account for the accelerated progression of atheroma in patients with diabetes. The adhesion molecules most involved in monocyte–endothelial cell interactions are intercellular adhesion molecule-1 (ICAM-1), vascular adhesion molecule-1 (VCAM-1) and E-selectin. High glucose levels up-regulate ICAM-1 protein and mRNA expression via a PKC-dependent pathway.

MEMBRANE TRANSPORT AND GLOMERULOPATHY

Expansion of the glomerular mesangium is an early feature of diabetic nephropathy, and isoform-specific translocation of PKC has been identified in glomerular cells. As well as increasing the synthesis of extracellular matrix components, PKC-mediated phosphorylation of the glomerular NA^+/K^+-ATPase affects cellular adhesion, vascular permeability and sodium–hydrogen transport. The activity of key membrane transporters, e.g. NA^+/K^+-ATPase and Ca^{2+}-ATPase, is reduced in diabetes, in part via PKC activation.

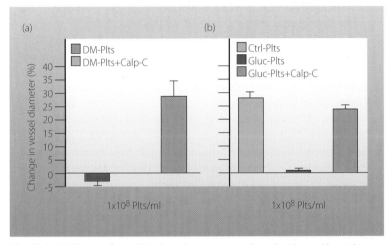

Fig. 19.4 (a) Platelets from diabetic patients were incubated with or without the PKC inhibitor, calphostin C, prior to being perfused through a normal rabbit carotid artery. Untreated diabetic platelets induce no vasodilator response, but platelet-mediated vasodilation was restored by treating diabetic platelets with a PKC inhibitor. (b) Similarly, platelets from non-diabetic subjects were incubated under normal or high glucose conditions. Treatment with high glucose impaired platelet-mediated vasodilation, but this was restored by treatment with the PKC inhibitor Adapted from *Br J Pharmacol* 1999; **127**: 903–8.

CURRENT ISSUES

- Hyperglycaemia, via isoform-selective PKC activation, affects a variety of pathophysiological pathways involved in the structural and functional abnormalities associated with diabetic vascular complications. These mechanisms are incompletely understood, but PKC activation influences gene expression, endothelial and VSM function and various cell membrane transporters.

- PKC-mediated stimulation of gene expression, particularly VPF and TGFβ formation, involves activation of the MAP kinase pathway and interaction with specific binding sites and transcription factors.

- Some of the therapeutic protection conferred by angiotensin-converting enzyme inhibitors (ACE-Is) and experimental compounds such as aminoguanadine may, in part, be mediated via reductions in tissue PKC activities.

- Activation of the calcium-dependent PKC isoforms, especially PKC-β, plays the most important role in mediating the diverse unwanted effects of PKC activation in vascular tissues.

FURTHER READING

Chan NN, Vallance P, Colhoun HM. Nitric oxide and vascular responses in type 1 diabetes. *Diabetologia* 2000; **43**: 137–47.

Idris I, Gray S, Donnnelly R. Protein kinase C activation: isozime-specific effects on metabolism and cardiovascular complications in diabetes. *Diabetologia* 2001; **44**: 659–673.

Inoguchi T, Li P, Umeda F et al. High glucose level and free fatty acid stimulate reactive oxygen species production through PKC-dependent activation of NADPH oxidase in cultured vascular cells. *Diabetes* 2000; **49**: 1939–45.

Oskarsson HJ, Hofmeyer TG, Coppey L, Yorek MA. Effect of protein kinase C and phospholipase A$_2$ inhibitors on the impaired ability of human diabetic platelets to cause vasodilation. *Br J Pharmacol* 1999; **127**: 903–8.

Tesfamariam B, Brown ML, Cohen RA. Elevated glucose impairs endothelium-dependent relaxation by activating protein kinase C. *J Clin Invest* 1991; **87**: 1643–8.

Williams B, Schrier RW. Characterization of glucose-induced *in situ* protein kinase C activity in cultured vascular smooth muscle cells. *Diabetes* 1992; **41**: 1464–72.

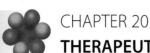

CHAPTER 20

Richard Donnelly MD, PhD, FRCP, FRACP

THERAPEUTIC POTENTIAL FOR ISOFORM-SELECTIVE PROTEIN KINASE C INHIBITORS

INTRODUCTION

Because protein kinase C (PKC) plays a fundamental role in normal pathways of cellular signal transduction, conventional thinking would suggest that a pharmacological inhibitor of PKC is unlikely to be a feasible option for clinical drug development. More recently, however, realization that PKC is a multifunctional family of isoenzymes with different patterns of tissue distribution, regulation and biochemical structure has led to renewed interest in the therapeutic potential of isoform-selective blockade of PKC activation, e.g. using antisense oligonucleotides or macrocyclic bis-indolylmaleimide compounds.

DISCOVERY OF LY333531—AN ORALLY ACTIVE AND HIGHLY SPECIFIC PKC-β INHIBITOR

First and second generation PKC inhibitors, such as the staurosporine-like compounds and isoquinolinesulphonamides (e.g. GF109203X), block the catalytic domain of PKC, which carries a high degree of sequence homologuey with other kinases, and are therefore non-specific for PKC.

George King's group at the Joslyn Diabetes Centre in Boston, USA, collaborating with scientists at Eli Lilly, undertook an extensive screening program to identify and optimize a PKC-β-selective inhibitor. The drug discovery programme was initiated on the basis of numerous experimental studies showing that hyperglycaemia-induced PKC activation involves predominantly PKC-β in retinal, glomerular and vascular tissues. LY333531, a bis-indolylmaleimide compound, was discovered in the early 1990s (**Fig. 20.1**). The selectivity for PKC-β relative to other PKC isoforms, and indeed other intracellular kinases, was clearly documented (**Table 20.1**). LY333531 inhibits PKC-β_I and PKC-β_{II} with half-maximal inhibitory constants (IC_{50}) of 4.7 and 5.9 nmol/l, respectively, whereas for other PKC isoenzymes (except PKC-η) the IC_{50} was 250 nmol/l or greater (**Table 20.1**). Thus, the compound has a unique profile of isoform selectivity.

The pharmacological effects of LY333531 have been evaluated successfully in numerous experimental models of diabetic microangiopathy, and this compound is now progressing into the late stages of full clinical development.

EFFECTS OF LY333531 IN DIABETIC RETINOPATHY

Hyperglycaemia-induced PKC activation increases retinal vascular permeability factor (VPF) gene expression and peptide synthesis, which markedly increases retinal endothelial permeability and also plays an important role in

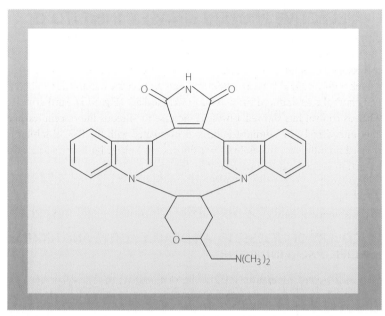

Fig. 20.1   Structure of LY333531, a macrocyclic bis-indolylmaleimide, which is an orally active, selective PKC-β inhibitor.

Tabulated IC$_{50}$ values for LY333531		
	IC$_{50}$ (nM)	
Kinase	**LY333531**	**Staurosporine**
PKC-α	360	45
PKC-β$_1$	4.7	23
PKC-β$_2$	5.9	19
PKC-γ	300	110
PKC-δ	250	28
PKC-ε	600	18
PKC-ζ	>10^5	>1.5×10^3
PKC-η	52	5
Cyclic AMP kinase	>10^5	100
Ca^{2+}-calmodulin kinase	8×10^3	4
Casein kinase	>10^5	1.4×10^4
Src tyrosine kinase	>10^5	1

Table 20.1 Tabulated IC$_{50}$ values (i.e. concentrations in nM required to achieve 50% inhibition of enzyme activity) for LY333531 and the non-specific PKC inhibitor, staurosporine, with respect to each PKC isoform and related intracellular kinases. Adapted from *Science* 1996; **472:** 728–31.

new vessel formation. Thus, blocking VPF-mediated retinal permeability is a prime target for therapeutic amelioration of diabetic maculopathy.

Studies in rats have clearly shown that intravitreal administration of VPF increases vitreous fluorescein leakage, and that pretreatment of these animals for 1 week with LY333531 25 mg/kg/day via oral administration ameliorated VPF and phorbol ester-induced vitreous fluorescein leakage (**Fig. 20.2**). Furthermore, whereas control rats showed a twofold increase in vitreous fluorescein leakage after intravitreal VPF administration, rats pretreated with the PKC-β inhibitor showed no difference in basal vitreous fluorescein leakage but there was a 96% reduction in VPF-induced vitreous fluorescein leakage (**Fig. 20.2**).

Increased retinal permeability is a hallmark of neovascularization within the diabetic eye, as well as being a sight-threatening pathological entity even in the absence of new vessel formation. These experimental data have shown that oral administration of LY333531 is well tolerated and considerably atten-

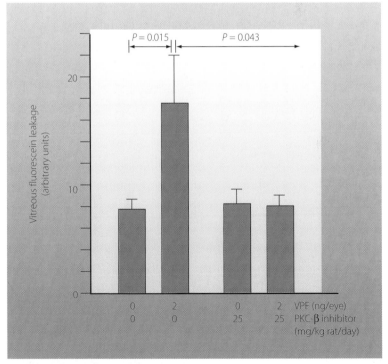

Fig. 20.2   Oral administration of the PKC-β inhibitor, LY333531, to normal rats prevents the increase in vitreous fluorescein leakage following intravitreal injection of VPF. Adapted from *Diabetes* 1997; **46**: 1473–1480.

uates VPF-mediated retinal permeability. Furthermore, diabetes is characterized by an increase in retinal mean circulation time (MCT), and oral treatment with LY333531 for 2 weeks in STZ-diabetic rats reduced retinal MCT,
as measured by video fluorescein angiography (**Fig. 20.3**). This experimental
data has now been confirmed in phase II clinical trials in which LY333531
administration for 1 month produced significant improvements in retinal
blood flow and MCT among 27 diabetic patients. Larger, multicentre clinical
trials are in progress.

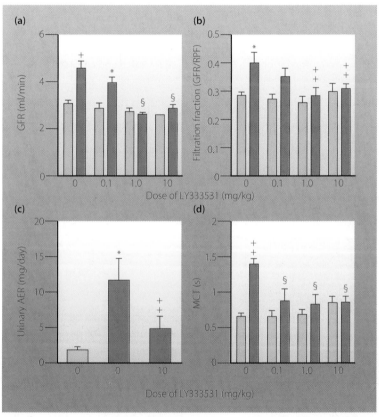

Fig. 20.3 Effect of oral dosing with LY333531 on renal and retinal vascular function
(RVS) in non-diabetic (●) and STZ-diabetic (●) rats. Untreated diabetic animals show
increases in glomerular filtration rate (GFR), renal filtration fraction (GFR corrected for
renal plasma flow, RPF), urinary albumin excretion rate (AER) and retinal mean
circulation time (MCT). Oral treatment with LY333531 0.1–10 mg/kg/day ameliorated
these renal and retinal haemodynamic abnormalities. *Science* 1996; **272**: 728–31.

Further experimental studies have shown that diabetes-induced reductions in Na^+/K^+-ATPase and Ca^{2+}-ATPase in the retina are mediated, in part, via PKC-β activation. Oral administration of LY333531 normalizes Na^+/K^+-ATPase activity in retinal microvessels (**Fig. 20.4**).

PKC-β INHIBITION AND EXPERIMENTAL NEPHROPATHY

The early stages of diabetic renal disease are characterized by glomerular hyperfiltration, mesangial expansion and microalbuminuria. Hyperglycaemia-induced *de novo* synthesis of DAG, coupled with activation of PKC, especially PKC-β, affects the structural and functional changes in the kidney via several different mechanisms involving various phosphorylation substrates of PKC. For example, mesangial expansion has been attributed, in part, to PKC-mediated increases in transforming growth factor-β (TGF-β) gene expression, activation of cytosolic phospholipase A_2 and inhibition of Na^+/K^+-ATPase activity.

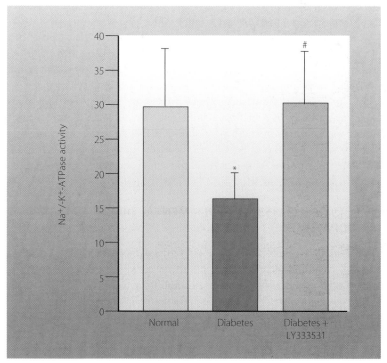

Fig. 20.4   Oral treatment with the PKC-β inhibitor LY333531, reverses diabetes-related reductions in Na^+/K^+-ATPase activity in retinal microvessels. Adapted from Kowluru *et al. Diabetes* 1998; **47**: 464–9.

Experimental studies with LY333531 have shown that, following oral administration for 8 weeks to STZ-diabetic and non-diabetic rats, urinary albumin excretion rate (AER) and glomerular hyperfiltration were significantly reduced (**Fig. 20.3**). Interestingly, higher doses of the PKC-β inhibitor (1–10 mg/kg/day) were required to inhibit diabetes-mediated PKC activation in the kidney compared with the retina (0.1 mg/kg/day). In addition, treatment with LY333531 had no significant effect on GFR and filtration fraction in non-diabetic animals (**Fig. 20.3**). Among diabetic rats, however, the dose–response curve for LY333531 in normalizing GFR paralleled its inhibitory effect on PKC activity.

Renal protection with aminoguanidine and angiotensin-converting enzyme (ACE) inhibition involves normalization of glomerular PKC activity

In experimental models of diabetic renal disease, e.g. the STZ-diabetic rat, it is well established that ACE-Is and aminoguanidine retard the structural and functional abnormalities characteristic of diabetic nephropathy, particularly with respect to reducing urinary AER. The exact mechanisms by which these therapeutic interventions work is not entirely clear, but recent work by George Jerums and colleagues has shown that glomerular PKC activity levels are normalized in STZ-diabetic rats during experimental treatment with aminoguanidine and the ACE-I, ramipril. Thus, diabetes-related increases in glomerular PKC activity may serve as an important common pathway by which metabolic and haemodynamic factors contribute to the initiation and progression of diabetic renal disease. Existing renoprotective agents, e.g. ACE-I, may slow the progression of nephropathy, in part, by normalizing diabetes-induced increases in glomerular PKC activity.

EFFECTS OF LY333531 IN EXPERIMENTAL DIABETIC NEUROPATHY

Various pathways have been implicated in the pathogenesis of diabetic neuropathy, including increased polyol pathway activity, enhanced non-enzymatic glycation and PKC activation. In addition, neural ischaemia is thought to play an important role in diabetic nerve injury, in part via PKC activation which impairs vasodilation and increases vasoconstrictor pathways in the endoneurial microvasculature.

In experimental STZ-diabetic rats, motor nerve conduction velocity and sciatic nerve blood flow are reduced. Treatment with the PKC-β inhibitor, LY333531, ameliorated these abnormalities via mechanisms attributable to prevention of neural ischaemia.

CLINICAL IMPLICATIONS OF AN ORALLY ACTIVE PKC-β INHIBITOR, LY333531

Extensive experimental studies have shown that LY333531 selectively inhibits PKC-β in retinal, renal and vascular tissues following oral administration without any significant adverse effects. The encouraging tolerability profile of LY333531 is no doubt attributable to its pharmacological specificity for PKC-β_I and PKC-β_{II}. The animal studies have convincingly shown that, following chronic oral treatment, LY333531 ameliorates the early increases in retinal blood flow, glomerular filtration rate and renal and retinal permeability.

These data open the possibility of a new and exciting pathway for therapeutic intervention in the earliest stages of diabetic microvascular disease. In particular, such an approach would be unique in offering protection against the development and progression of retinopathy and nephropathy via a mechanism that is independent of (and complementary to) glucose or blood pressure reduction. Thus, in clinical practice, PKC-β inhibition would be used as an adjunct to all existing therapies for the prevention of diabetic vascular complications. Large multicentre clinical trials are on-going not only in diabetic retinopathy and renal disease but also in patients with other diabetic complications, e.g. erectile dysfunction and diabetic neuropathy.

CURRENT ISSUES

* LY333531 is a unique orally active PKC inhibitor which is highly specific for the PKC-β isoforms. Following oral administration to STZ-diabetic rats, LY333531 prevented diabetes-related increases in retinal and renal PKC activity in parallel with amelioration of glomerular hyperfiltration, microalbuminuria and increased retinal blood flow.
* LY333531 shows an excellent tolerability profile in experimental diabetic animals, no doubt reflecting its specificity for inhibiting only two out of 12 PKC isoforms. Furthermore, in non-diabetic animals (in which there is no augmentation of PKC activity) LY333531 has no significant effects on retinal or renal haemodynamics. Thus, the compound seems to be highly specific for PKC-β and only achieves therapeutic effects in experimental studies in which diabetes-related increases in PKC are present.
* Large multicentre clinical trials with LY333531 are on-going to access its efficacy and safety in patients with diabetic retinopathy, and in due course further studies will be established to define the role of this compound in other diabetes complications, including nephropathy, erectile dysfunction and peripheral neuropathy.

FURTHER READING

Aiello LP, Bursell SE, Clermont A *et al.* Vascular endothelial growth factor-induced retinal permeability is mediated by protein kinase C *in vivo* and suppressed by an orally effective β-isoform-selective inhibitor. *Diabetes* 1997; **46**: 1473–80.

Ishii H, Jirousek MR, Koya D *et al.* Amelioration of vascular dysfunction in diabetic rats by an oral PKC-β inhibitor. *Science* 1996; **272**: 728–31.

Kowluru RA, Jirousek MR, Stramm L *et al.* Abnormalities of retinal metabolism in diabetes or experimental galactosemia: V relationship between protein kinase C and ATPase. *Diabetes* 1998; **47**: 464–9.

Nakamura J, Kato K, Hamada Y *et al.* A protein kinase C-β-selective inhibitor ameliorates neural dysfunction in streptozotocin-induced diabetic rats. *Diabetes* 1999; **48**: 2090–5.

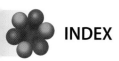

INDEX